Caring for Dependent Older Persons

CARING FOR DEPENDENT OLDER PERSONS

Jit Seng Tan • Shing Yuen Teo
Lotus Eldercare Pte Ltd, Singapore

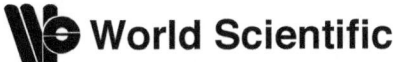

NEW JERSEY · LONDON · SINGAPORE · BEIJING · SHANGHAI · HONG KONG · TAIPEI · CHENNAI · TOKYO

Published by

World Scientific Publishing Co. Pte. Ltd.

5 Toh Tuck Link, Singapore 596224

USA office: 27 Warren Street, Suite 401-402, Hackensack, NJ 07601

UK office: 57 Shelton Street, Covent Garden, London WC2H 9HE

Library of Congress Cataloging-in-Publication Data
Names: Tan, Jit Seng, author. | Teo, Shing Yuen, author.
Title: Caring for dependent older persons / Jit Seng Tan, Lotus Eldercare Pte Ltd,
 Singapore, Shing Yuen Teo, Lotus Eldercare Pte Ltd, Singapore.
Description: New Jersey : World Scientific, 2018. | Includes index.
Identifiers: LCCN 2018035628 | ISBN 9789813239999 (pbk. : alk. paper)
Subjects: LCSH: Older people--Care. | Geriatric nursing.
Classification: LCC RC954 .T34 2018 | DDC 618.97/0231--dc23
LC record available at https://lccn.loc.gov/2018035628

British Library Cataloguing-in-Publication Data
A catalogue record for this book is available from the British Library.

Copyright © 2019 by World Scientific Publishing Co. Pte. Ltd.

All rights reserved. This book, or parts thereof, may not be reproduced in any form or by any means, electronic or mechanical, including photocopying, recording or any information storage and retrieval system now known or to be invented, without written permission from the publisher.

For photocopying of material in this volume, please pay a copying fee through the Copyright Clearance Center, Inc., 222 Rosewood Drive, Danvers, MA 01923, USA. In this case permission to photocopy is not required from the publisher.

For any available supplementary material, please visit
https://www.worldscientific.com/worldscibooks/10.1142/10983#t=suppl

Typeset by Stallion Press
Email: enquiries@stallionpress.com

Preface

Having cared for many dependent older persons long term in their own homes as their physician in charge, I am very privileged to have worked with many tireless caregivers. No matter whether they are formal carers like foreign domestic workers or informal ones like spouse, children or family, I have learnt much and am still learning from their innovative and effective ways in caring for their dependent elders.

Caring for dependent older person is a 24/7 work, which only the most tenacious individuals can withstand the journey. I am happy to know some of these very inspiring carers and dedicate this book to all of them.

There are many more detailed and "heavier" caregiver guides and books, written by experts, mine serves more as a breadth of the topics rather than the depth needed in caring for a dependent older person.

I hope it will be a useful guide in helping carers in their various care giving journey.

Dr. Tan Jit Seng
August 2018

Acknowledgements

We would like to thank the following companies for their generosity in allowing us to share their products/photos.

- Lifeline Corporation Pte. Ltd. for the rehabilitation equipment photos
- Mr Seng Ian Hao and Miss Seng Ing Le from QaneMate, for the QaneMate photos
- Mr Michael Pang from Winner SG, for the transfer wheelchair photo
- Tukimed Ltd. and Mr Jussi Peltonen from HoviCare, for the Wheelator photo
- ConvaTec for the wound products photos
- ExoAtlet Asia for the exoskeleton photo
- TUV SUD for the photo of telemonitoring screens
- Ohmni Labs for the photo of a telepresence robot
- Nucleus Dynamics for the photos of NDKare
- Pastel Health for the photo of Chatbotsforhealth

We would also like to thank Ms Lynette Chan, speech therapist from LC Speech Therapy, for her help in reviewing parts of our book.

Contents

Preface v
Acknowledgements vi

1. Introduction 1

    Aging Population Trend 1
    Activities of Daily Living (ADLs) 2

2. Training Modules for the Caregiver of a Dependent Older Person 5

    Module 1: Basic Care of a Dependent Older Person 5
    Module 2: Health Index Monitoring at Home 21
    Module 3: Food, Medication and Supplement Administration 27
    Module 4: Equipment Management 34
    Module 5: Home Environment Assessment, Rehabilitation
       and Infection Control 39
    Module 6: Basic Wound Management and Dressing 42
    Module 7: Recognition of Emergent Conditions 46

3. Effects of Aging and Common Diseases 49

    Part 1: Effects of Aging 49
    Part 2: Common Diseases Encountered by Caregivers 51

4. Caregiver Stress Management 61

    How to Identify Caregiver Stress? 63
    Different Caregiver Stress in Different Clinical Situations 64

5. Financial Support and Useful Information for Eldercare 69

    Part 1: Financial Subsidies 69
    Part 2: Lasting Power of Attorney (LPA) 82

Part 3: Appointment of a Deputy for an Older Person
  Lacking Mental Capacity 83
Part 4: Useful Information for Eldercare 84

6. Current and Future Technologies Supporting Eldercare 85

Types and Uses of Technologies 85
Examples of Current New Technologies and Future
  Technologies 87

Index 93

1 Introduction

AGING POPULATION TREND

According to the Department of Statistics, Singapore, the percentage of Singapore residents above 65 years of age was 13% in 2017. The percentage had risen over the years, from 6% in 1990 to 10.5% in 2013, and to 13% in 2017.

The ratio of residents (as shown in Table 1 and Chart 1 from the Department of Statistics, Singapore) aged 20–64 to residents aged 65 and above continued to fall from 6.7 in 2012 to 5.1 in 2017. Thus, there will be fewer younger persons to support each older person in years to come.

Table 1. Age Distribution of Singapore Resident Population.

Age Group (Years)	1990	2000	2010	2012	2013	2016	2017
Below 15	23.0%	21.9%	17.4%	16.4%	16.0%	15.2%	15.0%
15–24	16.9%	12.9%	13.5%	13.7%	13.6%	12.7%	12.4%
25–34	21.5%	17.0%	15.1%	14.4%	14.4%	14.4%	14.4%
35–44	16.9%	19.4%	16.7%	16.3%	16.1%	15.6%	15.4%
45–54	9.0%	14.3%	16.6%	16.5%	16.4%	15.7%	15.5%
55–64	6.7%	7.2%	11.7%	12.7%	13.1%	14.0%	14.2%
65 & Over	6.0%	7.2%	9.0%	9.9%	10.5%	12.4%	13.0%

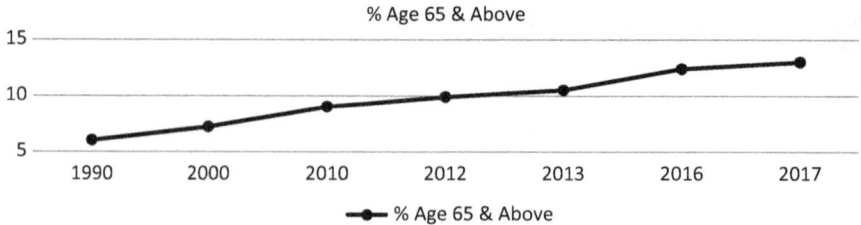

Chart 1. Percentage of Residents Aged 65 and Above Over the Years.

ACTIVITIES OF DAILY LIVING (ADLS)

ADLs are the things that we routinely do, without needing assistance. The activities include washing or bathing, dressing, feeding, toileting, transferring and mobility. An older person may have reduced ability to perform ADLs, owing to functional decline in aging or to a chronic health problem. A decrease in ADLs is most drastically felt after a major illness such as a stroke or even after a serious infection for an older person. The purpose of assessing the person's ability to perform ADLs is to provide objective data for observing improvement or decline in the health status and for planning the care of the person.

The Basic ADLs are:

(1) *Washing or bathing*
    The ability to wash in the bath or shower (including getting into and out of the bath or shower) or to wash by other means.
(2) *Dressing*
    The ability to put on, take off, secure and unfasten all garments (upper and lower) and, as appropriate, any braces, artificial limbs or other surgical or medical appliances.
(3) *Feeding*
    The ability to feed oneself food after it has been prepared and made available.
(4) *Toileting*
    The ability to use the lavatory or manage bowel and bladder function through the use of protective undergarments or surgical appliances if appropriate.

(5) *Mobility*
    The ability to move indoors from room to room on level surfaces.
(6) *Transferring*
    The ability to move from a bed to a chair or wheelchair, and vice versa.

The ability to perform ADLs is a common gauge of disabilities for insurance claims. A person will be eligible for claims if he or she is unable to perform at least three of the ADLs.

In 2012, there were 27,900 Singapore residents above the age of 60 with at least one ADL limitation needing assistance. However, there were only 10,692 beds in intermediate and long-term care facilities.

By 2030, it is projected that there will be 57,300 Singapore residents above the age of 60 with at least one ADL limitation needing assistance. Of these residents, it has been projected that 48,000 (83%) will reside at home. This coupled with the decrease in the ratio of younger persons supporting older persons means that the burden of caring for the old in Singapore is increasing.

To provide good care for the dependent older persons at home, we will need to train the caregivers. The caregivers will be empowered and have the knowledge to provide a good quality of care to the dependent older persons. There is also a lesser chance of the caregivers getting caregiver stress if they know what to expect and what to do. The dependent older person will also face fewer problems with good care from the caregiver. In addition, is better for the dependent older person to stay in an environment that he or she is familiar with.

A trained caregiver will be able to help the older person with the ADLs and to monitor the health of the older person. The caregiver should be able to identify if the older person is unwell and start simple treatment if needed or to sound the alarm for more help. In this case, the trained caregiver will be able to decrease the morbidity and mortality of the older person.

With better-trained caregivers, dependent older persons can get more professional care at home and prevent reversible conditions, for example constipation leading to complications such as urosepsis requiring hospitalisation for more invasive treatment.

2 Training Modules for the Caregiver of a Dependent Older Person

MODULE 1: BASIC CARE OF A DEPENDENT OLDER PERSON

Part 1: Washing/Bathing

Performance Skill #1: Proper Hand Washing Techniques

Step 1: Wet your hands and apply soap. Rub the palms together.
Step 2: Rub the back of both hands.
Step 3: Interlace the fingers and rub the hands together.
Step 4: Interlock the fingers and rub the back of the fingers of both hands together.
Step 5: Rub the thumb in a rotating manner, then the area between the index finger and the thumb, for both hands.
Step 6: Rub the fingertips on the palm for both hands.
Step 7: Rub both wrists in a rotating manner. Rinse and dry the hands thoroughly.

Performance Skill #2: Partial Bed Bath/Full Shower or Tub Bath

Partial Bed Bath

Step 1: Inform the older person about the bath and ensure privacy.
Step 2: Make sure that the temperature of the bathing water is lukewarm and comfortable.

Step 3: Wipe the face (eye area first) and progress down to the arm, chest and back, pelvis and gluteal area, and finally the lower limbs. Clean the washcloth after wiping each different body part or use a new bathing wipe. Use dry shampoo for the hair if needed.

Step 4: Dry the person and apply moisturiser over the body and barrier cream to the diaper areas.

Step 5: Change the linen if necessary.

Full Shower or Tub Bath

Step 1: Transfer the older person safely via a commode to the shower room.

Step 2: Ensure that the temperature of the bathing water is lukewarm and comfortable.

Step 3: Wash the face first with mild soap, followed by the rest of the body. Use soft white paraffin as soap if needed.

Step 4: Dry the person and apply moisturiser over the body and barrier cream to the diaper areas.

Step 5: Change the linen if necessary.

Performance Skill #3: Performing Shaving and Nail Care

Performing Shaving

Step 1: Clean the area, before shaving, with lukewarm water.

Step 2: Apply shaving cream if available.

Step 3: Shave the beard on the face (cheeks/upper lips/chin) in the direction of hair growth.

Step 4: Shave the beard on the neck against the direction of hair growth.

Step 5. Clean and dry the shaven areas. Apply aftershave lotion if available.

Nail Care

Step 1: Clean the foot and nails (outside and inside) with lukewarm water, and mild soap if needed.

Step 2: If the nails are thick, soak the foot in lukewarm water for 10–15 min before attempting to trim the nails.

Step 3: Trim the nails straight across with toenail clippers; do not cut inwards at the corners.

Step 4: Clean and dry the nails, and apply foot lotion if available.

Performance Skill #4: Maintaining Oral Hygiene

Step 1: Clean the oral cavity with gauze dampened in clean water or a non-alcohol mouthwash (e.g. Oral 7®), or sodium bicarbonate oral swabs if available.

Step 2: Clean the teeth with a soft bristled toothbrush at least two times a day.

Step 3: Apply oral gels like Oral 7® moisturising gel for dry oral cavity if needed.

Part 2: Dressing

Performance Skill #5: Upper Body Dressing

Step 1: Choose comfortable loose clothing or adaptive clothing if available.

Step 2: Sit the older person up if possible, instead of lying or standing.

Step 3: Dress the weaker or more dependent side first, owing to possible stiffness or spasticity and less flexibility than the non-affected side.

Step 4: Allow the person to button the clothing on his or her own if possible, as a form of occupational therapy.

Performance Skill #6: Lower Body Dressing

Step 1: Choose comfortable loose clothing; consider the use of adaptive clothing or a *sarong* for easy dressing.

Step 2: Lay the older person down and flex the knees to start putting on the trousers.

Step 3: Turn the person from side to side to pull up the trousers to the waist level.

Part 3: Feeding

Performance Skill #7: Oral Feeding — Spoon

Step 1: Ensure that the dependent older person is alert before feeding.

Step 2: Ensure that the food is at a comfortable temperature for eating (avoid food that is too hot or too cold).

Step 3: Proper positioning of the person: sit him or her upright and with the neck slightly flexed and the chin down, for the optimum position to swallow.

Step 4: Feed the person at a comfortable pace, and check the oral cavity for completion of swallowing before starting to feed the next spoonful. *DO NOT RUSH*. Expect the feeding process to take at least 30–60 min.

Step 5: Monitor for signs of choking, such as cough, breathlessness or the lips and face turning blue, during the feeding.

Step 6: After the feeding, check the oral cavity again for any residue and keep the person at least 45 degrees upright for the next 30–90 min. Avoid laying him or her down, to prevent regurgitation of the meal.

Performance Skill #8: Oral Feeding — Syringe

Syringe feeding is unlikely to be appropriate. Consult professionals if the family is using syringes to feed the dependent older person.

Performance Skill #9: Preparing Fluids of Different Consistencies

Step 1: There are three thickened fluid consistencies: pudding-thickened (thickest), honey-thickened and nectar-thickened (least thick) fluid. Confirm which one is recommended by the speech therapist after a swallowing assessment.

Step 2: For the consistency required, follow the instructions on the can of thickener regarding the ratio of thickener to fluid needed. For example, to prepare honey-thickened fluids using Resource® Clear thickener, use two level scoops of thickener powder to 100 mL of water or other fluid.

Step 3: Stir vigorously when the thickener is added to the fluid, to dissolve it. Let the thickened fluid sit for 5 min, then stir again before serving.

Performance Skill #10: Preparing Solids of Different Consistencies

Step 1: Modified solids include a blended diet, a minced diet and a soft diet.
Step 2: For a blended diet, all foods (e.g. porridge, vegetables, meats) have to be processed in a blender until a smooth puree is achieved.

For a minced diet, certain foods, such as Chinese vegetables, can be processed in a blender or chopper until a "minced" consistency is achieved. This diet can also include porridge, minced meat, finely flaked pieces of fish and other soft vegetables (e.g. steamed broccoli) that can be easily broken up into smaller pieces with the back of a fork.

For a soft diet, all foods have to be soft in texture (e.g. porridge, soft rice, well-stewed meats, soft vegetables) and easily broken apart with a fork.

Performance Skill #11: Nasogastric Tube Feeding and Management

Step 1: Determine whether the nasogastric tube is a temporary Ryles tube (PVC) to be changed in 2 weeks or a more lasting Corflo or Kangaroo tube (medical grade polyurethane) to be changed in 2–3 months.
Step 2: Recognise the size of the tube — either 12F or 14F — from the marking on the tube feeding ports. Do note that smaller or larger tubes are also available but are less commonly used.
Step 3: Measure the exposed length of the tube to determine the correct length of the tube inserted.
Step 4: Know the methods of securing the tube at the nose with the use of tapes, e.g. 3M Micropore Medical Tape. Change the tape every 2–3 days.

Method 1: Using a ½-inch tape

- Cut a 10 cm length of tape.
- Stick one end to the tip of the nostril.
- Wind the other end around the nasogastric tube and then stick that end to the tip of the nose.
- Stick a 3–4 cm tape to the plastered ends to further secure the tube.

Method 2: Using a 1-inch tape

- Cut a 5–7 cm length of tape.
- Cut into the middle of the tape, leaving a 2–3 cm portion.
- Stick the uncut portion of the tape to the tip of the nostril.
- Wind the two cut "tails" around the tube in different directions.

Step 5: Prepare the milk feed and water flush.

- Know the volume of milk to be fed and the timings.
- Use the milk feed at room temperature, or slightly lukewarm if the family is keen.
- Know the volume of water to be flushed at the end of the feed.
- Feed no more than 400 mL per bolus session, to prevent sudden over-inflation and regurgitation.

Step 6: Check the placement of the tube before feeding.

- Measure the exposed length of the tube.
- Aspirate from the tube for any remnant undigested milk and gastric fluid.
- Test the aspirate with the pH indicator; if the pH is around 2–4, it is safe to feed. If the older person is on medications to reduce production of gastric acids, the pH may be around 5–6.
- Check the content of the aspirates. It can be a clear yellowish gastric juice or a thicker milky aspirate.
- Take note of the volume. If it is less than half the volume of the normal feeds, discard the aspirate and resume normal feeding.
- If the volume is more than half the volume of the normal feeds, put back the aspirate and skip the current intended feed. Check again when the next feed is due.
- Always flush the tube with the pre-instructed volume of water, to prevent tube clogging.

Step 7: Monitor for signs of choking, such as cough, breathlessness or the lips and face turning blue, during the feeding.

Step 8: Keep the person at least 30–45 degrees upright for at least 1 hr after the feeding.

Step 9: Take note when the nasogastric tube is due for a change, and arrange for the tube to be changed.

Note

For an older person on a continuous feeding pump, check the feeding bag and the setting of the pump. Hospitals routinely start with 10–40 mL an hour, upping the rate by 10–20 mL an hour until the desired volume and calories of the nutrition are achieved. The duration may range from 8 to 20 hr per day, depending on the person's condition.

Performance Skill #12: Percutaneous Endoscopic Gastrostomy (PEG) Tube Feeding and Management

Step 1: Check the placement of the PEG tube by the marking at the abdominal stoma, usually at 2–4 cm.

Step 2: Check for leaks around the PEG stoma before feeding.

Step 3: Prepare the milk feed and water flush.

- Know the volume of milk to be fed and the timings.
- Use the milk feed at room temperature, or lukewarm if the family is keen.
- Know the volume of water to be flushed at the end of the feed.

Step 4: Open the feeding port and connect it to the feeding syringe.

Step 5: Feed the older person while taking care of any leaks around the stoma site upon feeding.

Part 4: Toileting

Performance Skill #13: Changing Diapers and Applying Barrier Cream

Step 1: The frequency of diaper change is about every 3–5 hr, depending on the older person's bowel condition. Normal diaper usage can be about 2 (for those with indwelling catheters) to 8 diapers a day.

Step 2: Always clean the perineal area in the front-to-back direction once for each clean wipe, in one smooth motion. Use more wet hospital wipes if needed; do not reuse a once wipe it has been soiled.

Step 3: Always use barrier cream on the diaper areas of the skin for each diaper change, to prevent excoriation of the skin in contact with wetted diapers.

Performance Skill #14: Changing Urine Bags and Managing Urinary Catheters

Step 1: An older person with an indwelling catheter should have his or her urinary bag changed by the caregiver once or twice a week.

Step 2: Clean both hands, and wear gloves if possible.

Step 3: Clean the connection between the urinary catheter and the urine bag with an alcohol swab before disengaging. Bend the catheter before pulling out the connector, to prevent urine leakage.

Step 4: Not touching the tip of the connector, push the tip of the new urine bag into the catheter port.

Step 5: Ensure that the outlet of the catheter is not touching the floor, and always avoid placing the urine bag higher than the person's body, to prevent urine from flowing back into the urinary bladder.

Step 6: Similarly, when draining the urine bag, wash your hands, and wear a glove if possible.

Step 7: Use an alcohol swab to clean the outlet port before pulling it open to drain out urine from the urine bag.

Step 8: Clean with a new alcohol swab again before pushing back the port to close the outlet.

Performance Skill #15: Maintaining Perineal Hygiene and Care

For Male Older Persons

Step 1: Pull the foreskin back to clean the areas around the glans penis, usually covered by the foreskin. Clean the areas over and around the scrotum sac.

Step 2: Always make sure that the foreskin is pulled forward covering the glans penis, to avoid the risk of getting paraphimosis.

Step 3: Use a separate washcloth or a new hospital wipe after each area or each wipe.

Step 4: Always keep the area clean and dry, and inform a health care professional if the area becomes red or develops scaly rashes.

For Female Older Persons

Step 1: Clean from outer to inner: from the labia majora to the labia minora, vagina and clitoris. Clean the labiafolds over the outer side and then the inner side, before gently exposing the labia with the non-dominant hand to expose the urethral meatus and vaginal orifice. Clean the exposed urethral meatus and vaginal orifice, and do not put pressure on the urinary catheter if present.

Step 2: Always move from the genital area to the perineum and then the anus, to avoid contamination.

Step 3: Use a separate washcloth or a new hospital wipe after each area or each swipe.

Step 4: Always keep the area clean and dry, and inform a health care professional if the area becomes red or develops scaly rashes.

Part 5: Transferring

Performance Skill #16a: Turning and Side-Lying Positions in Bed

Step 1: Inform the older person that you are about to turn him or her to his or her right/left side. In special circumstances, for example an older person with a craniectomy over the left side with a defect in the cranium, it would be best to turn the person always to his or her right to avoid pressure on the brain with a defective skull.
Step 2: Flex and internally rotate both shoulder joints to bring the upper limbs in front and well supported by the chest wall to avoid injuries to the limbs on turning.
Step 3: Slightly flex the knee joints before turning the person.
Step 4: Place one hand over the shoulder and the other over the hip joint for good support before turning the person towards you.
Step 5: A pillow can be placed under the person's back for support in that position.

Performance Skill #16b: Sitting the Older Person up from a Lying Position

Step 1: Inform the older person that you are about to sit him or her up on the bedside.
Step 2: Flex and internally rotate both shoulder joints to bring the upper limbs in front and well supported by the chest wall to avoid injuries to the limbs on turning.
Step 3: Slight flex the knee joints before turning the person.
Step 4: Bend forwards, hugging the person with one arm across the neck to the upper back on one side and over the hip to the buttock area on the other side.
Step 5: Ask the person to slowly lower his or her lower limbs down the bed, with you pulling over the hip area while pushing the body upright with your arm across the back.

Performance Skill #17a: Transferring from Bed to Chair/Commode

Step 1: Help the older person to sit up on the bed and if possible, lower the bed to a comfortable level, with both feet on the floor by the side.
Step 2: Shift the chair or commode at 45 degrees to the bed and place one hand of the person on the seat handle. Remember to lock the wheels of the wheelchair or commode after putting it in place.
Step 3: Ask the person to attempt to stand from sitting and to stand up at the count of 3, the while using the other hand to grip the belt or the clothing over the hip to stabilise him or her.
Step 4: Lift the person up and slowly ask him or her to rotate his or her body and sit down on the wheelchair or commode.

Performance Skill #17b: Transferring from Wheelchair to Bed or Vehicle

Step 1: Position the wheelchair at 45 degrees to the bed or vehicle.
Step 2: Lock the wheel of the wheelchair.
Step 3: Place the arms of the older person around the neck of the caregiver.
Step 4: Grip the person's belt or a transfer belt.
Step 5: Bend your knees slightly and pull the body of the person forwards, towards yourself.
Step 6: Instruct the older person to attempt standing at the count of 3, while you make the pull using the belt with each count.
Step 7: Slowly rotate the person's body with the back to the seat or bed, after getting him or her to stand upright.
Step 8: Allow the person to slowly be seated in the bed or vehicle.

Part 6: Mobility

Assessment by a physiotherapist is usually done to prescribe the correct walking aids to be used and the older person is taught the proper use of the devices.

Performance Skill #18: Identification of Different Types of Walking Aids

Walking stick		Different designs are available. Height-adjustable; some maybe foldable. Products shown are from Lifeline Corporation Pte. Ltd.
Crutches		Axillary crutch and elbow crutch. Height-adjustable. Different sizes available for children and adults. Products shown are from Lifeline Corporation Pte. Ltd.
Quad cane		2 versions: narrow base and broad base. Broad base one is more stable but more difficult for use on stairs. Product shown is from Lifeline Corporation Pte. Ltd.
Dual-purpose umbrella and walking stick		Product shown is from Lifeline Corporation Pte. Ltd.

QaneMate		Developed by 2 young Singaporeans, Seng Ian Hao (13 yr old) and his sister Seng Ing Le (11 yr old). Makes walking sticks safer and smarter. Product shown is from QaneMate.
Foldable walking frame		2 versions: fixed and reciprocal. Product shown is from Lifeline Corporation Pte. Ltd.
Foldable rising walking frame		Has a set of lower handgrips which user pushes against when rising from sitting position. Product shown is from Lifeline Corporation Pte. Ltd.
Foldable walking frame with front castors		2 versions: fixed and reciprocal. Product shown is from Lifeline Corporation Pte. Ltd.
Rollator-cum-pushchair		Product shown is from Lifeline Corporation Pte. Ltd.

| Wheelator | 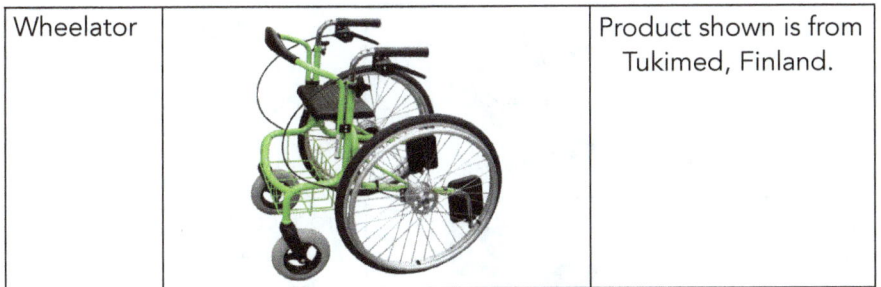 | Product shown is from Tukimed, Finland. |

Performance Skill #19: Identification of Different Types of Wheelchairs

Wheelchair		2 versions: standard and lightweight Product shown is from Lifeline Corporation Pte. Ltd.
Reclining wheelchair		Product shown is from Lifeline Corporation Pte. Ltd.
Lightweight pushchair		Wheels are small; older person will not be able to wheel himself/herself. Product shown is from Lifeline Corporation Pte. Ltd.
Transfer wheelchair		Winner Ultimate Wheelchair is designed, developed and made in Singapore. Rear wheel retractable, so easier to transfer older person. Product shown is from Winner SG.

Powered wheelchair		Product shown is from Lifeline Corporation Pte. Ltd.
Scooter		Product shown is from Lifeline Corporation Pte. Ltd.

Note: The products shown are examples and not an exhaustive list.

Performance Skill #20: Assisting the Ambulation of a Frail Older Person

Step 1: Sit the older person up by the side of the bed with the feet touching the ground and ask him or her for symptoms of light-headedness or giddiness.

Step 2: Use a walking or transfer belt if available.

Step 3: Have both upper limbs with the hand supporting the body on the edge of the bed.

Step 4: Stand in front of the person with both your feet blocking both his or her feet.

Step 5: Ask the person to prepare to stand from sitting and to stand up at the count of 3.

Step 6: Bend your knees slightly and request the person to lean towards you, with you keeping your back straight.

Step 7: At the count of 3, lift the your person up from a sitting position by pulling on the transfer belt, and co-ordinate with him or her the movement to stand upright.

Step 8: Allow the person to steady him or herself before initiating the walk.

Step 9: Hold firmly onto the belt and steady the person when he or she ambulates, and walk by his or her side.

MODULE 2: HEALTH INDEX MONITORING AT HOME

Performance Skill #21: Blood Pressure Monitoring Using a Manual Sphygmomanometer

Step 1: The older person sits and rests for 10–15 min first.
Step 2: The person rests the left arm on the table in front of him or her. The arm should be flexed and at the level of the heart.
Step 3: Wrap the cuff around the upper arm. The bottom edge of the cuff should be about 1 inch from the elbow. The cuff should be wrapped snugly, not too tight or too loose. You should be able to insert the tips of your fingers from the edge of the cuff.
Step 4: Place the wide head of the stethoscope against the skin on the inside of the arm. The edge of the diaphragm should be just beneath the cuff, positioned over the brachial artery.
Step 5: Gently put the earpieces of the stethoscope in your ears.
Step 6: Take the rubber bulb and tighten the valve.
Step 7: Rapidly squeeze the bulb to inflate the cuff to 180 mmHg.
Step 8: Slowly release the valve of the bulb to reduce air pressure from the cuff.
Step 9: Listen with the stethoscope while observing the sphygmomanometer. When you hear the first thumping or knocking sound, that is the systolic pressure. When the thumping or knocking sound disappears, that is the diastolic pressure.
Step 10: Record the blood pressure reading on the BP chart.

Performance Skill #22: Blood Pressure Monitoring Using Electronic Blood Pressure Machines

Step 1: The older person sits and rests for 10–15 min first.
Step 2: The person rests the left arm on the table in front of him or her. The arm should be flexed and at the level of the heart.
Step 3: Wrap the cuff around the upper arm. The bottom edge of the cuff should be about 1 inch from the elbow. The cuff should be wrapped snugly, not too tight or too loose. You should be able to insert the tips of your fingers from the edge of the cuff. The line from the cuff should point towards the middle finger.

Step 4: Switch on the blood pressure machine and press the "Start" button.
Step 5: The meter will auto-inflate the cuff and deflate it to get a reading.
Step 6: Record the blood pressure reading on the BP chart.

Blood Pressure Chart

Date	Time	Blood Pressure	Heart Rate
02/05/18	12.05 p.m.	139/80	60

Note: There are different cuff sizes available. Choose a cuff size that is suitable for the older person, an obese or muscular older person may need a bigger cuff.

Blood pressure is elevated after smoking, eating, or taking a drink with caffeine. Wait for 1 hr after these activities, then take the BP reading.

Performance Skill #23: Postural Blood Pressure Monitoring

Step 1: Have the older person lie down for 5 min. Take and record the blood pressure, heart rate, and associated symptoms if any.
Step 2: Have the person sit up. Take and record the blood pressure, heart rate, and associated symptoms if any.
Step 3: Have the person stand up. Take and record the blood pressure, heart rate, and associated symptoms if any.

Date: _____ Time: _____

Position	Time	Readings	Symptoms
Lying	5 min	BP ____/____ HR _____	
Sitting	1 min	BP ____/____ HR _____	
Standing	1 min	BP ____/____ HR _____	

Note: A drop in blood pressure of ≥20 mmHg, or in diastolic blood pressure of ≥10 mmHg, or experiencing light-headedness or dizziness is considered abnormal.

Performance Skill #24: Monitoring of the Pulse Rate

Step 1: Place the second and third fingertips on the inside of the wrist at the base of the thumb.
Step 2: Press lightly until you feel the pulse. Move to locate the pulse if needed.
Step 3: Look at a watch and count the beats in 1 min.
Step 4: Record the pulse rate.

Performance Skill #25: Monitoring of the Respiratory Rate

Step 1: The older person is at rest.
Step 2: Observe the rise and fall of the person's chest. One respiration is one complete rise and fall of the chest. Count the respirations in 1 min.
Step 3: Record the respiratory rate.

Performance Skill #26: Monitoring of the Temperature via a Digital Oral Thermometer

Step 1: Put the oral thermometer into a thermometer sleeve.
Step 2: Switch on the thermometer and wait till "L°C" is shown on the screen.
Step 3: Put the thermometer into the older person's mouth under the tongue. Close the mouth.
Step 4: Hold the thermometer in place till a beeping sound is heard.
Step 5: Take out the thermometer, and record the reading and the time of reading. Discard the thermometer sleeve.

Note

The person should not eat or drink anything 5 min before the temperature taking.

Performance Skill #27: Monitoring of the Temperature via an Ear Thermometer

Step 1: Put on a new probe cover for the ear thermometer.
Step 2: Press the "on" button of the thermometer.

Step 3: Pull the person's ear upwards and backwards. Put the tip of the probe into the ear; do not use force or push hard.
Step 4: Press the button and hold it till a long beep is heard.
Step 5: Take out the probe and record the reading.

Note

Different ear thermometers may have different procedures for taking the temperature. Refer to the instruction manual of your product for more details.

Performance Skill #28: Monitoring of Weight

Step 1: Ensure that the older person is standing well on the weighing scale and record the reading.

Date	Time	Weight
02/01/18	9 a.m.	50 kg
03/01/18	9 a.m.	50.5 kg

Note

Weighing chairs and bed scales are available for more dependent older persons.

Performance Skill #29: Monitoring of Oxygen Saturation via Pulse Oximetry

Step 1: Put the finger of the older person into the pulse oximeter, and it should power on and start to take a reading.
Step 3: Ensure that the bars indicating the heart rate are moving on the screen, showing that the meter is taking a reading. If the bars are not moving or only 1–2 bars are shown, change to another finger.
Step 4: Record the SpO_2, which is the oxygen saturation level and the heart rate.

Note

The finger of the person should be used and not the thumb. His or her fingers should not move about too much.

Performance Skill #30: Monitoring of Blood Capillary Glucose

Step 1: Wash both the older person's hand and your hands with soap and water. Dry the hands thoroughly.

Step 2: Unscrew the bottom of the lancing device. Insert a lancet and push it all the way in. Remove the top of the lancet to reveal the needle. Cap back the top of the lancing device. Prime the lancet, usually by pulling the end of the lancing device. Set the depth to which the needle will poke at level 1 or 2.

Step 3: Take out a test strip and insert into the blood glucose testing machine. The machine should power on and show a symbol of dropping blood.

Step 4: Place the lancing device to the side of the finger near the tip. Press the button.

Step 5: Squeeze the finger very gently to get a drop of blood. Apply the drop of blood to the test strip. Do note that for most machines the blood is usually sucked in from the side of the test strip.

Step 6: The machine starts running and a result is given. Record the result.

Step 7: Unscrew the bottom of the lancing device and insert the needle into the top part of the lancet, which you have just removed. Eject the used lancet into the bin.

Note

As there are various models on the market, the instructions for each machine and lancing device may vary. Do refer to the instruction manual.

Always use the strips for the correct brand and model of blood glucose machine. Bring along the empty bottle when buying a new bottle of strips.

Be careful about the storage conditions of the strips. Never expose them to warm temperature.

Some brands of strips must be used within 2–3 mths of the first opening. Do check your strips if such a condition applies.

Date	Time	Before Food/Hours After Food	Reading in mmol/L
02/01/18	8 a.m.	Before food	5.0
02/01/18	2 p.m.	2 hr after food (porridge)	8.6

MODULE 3: FOOD, MEDICATION AND SUPPLEMENT ADMINISTRATION

Performance Skill #31a: Administration of Oral Medications

Step 1: If the older person is on many medications, use a pill box to group the medications into medicines to be taken in the morning, afternoon, night or before bedtime. Take care as to whether a medication is to be taken with or without food. Try to give the medications at the same time each day.

Step 2: Pour the person a cup of water and pass him or her the medications to be taken at that point of time. Ensure that the person takes all the medications.

Step 3: If the supply of medications is running low, i.e. there is only 2–3 weeks' supply left, inform the decision-maker or employer about it.

Step 4: If you forget to give the person the medications, do not panic. Give the medications as soon as you remember. However, if it is near to the next dose timing, forget about the missed dose and just give the next dose. Do NOT double the dose of medications.

Performance Skill #31b: Administration of Eye Drops/Eye Ointment/Eye Gel

Administration of Eye Drops

Step 1: Wash your hands with soap and water, then dry them.
Step 2: Gently shake the bottle of eye drops.
Step 3: Tilt the older person's head back.
Step 4: Pull the lower lid away from the eye using the index finger.
Step 5: Uncap the bottle and invert it above the eye and squeeze gently. Let one drop of the medicine enter the eye. Do not touch the dropper against the eyelid or anything else.
Step 6: Replace the cap of the bottle immediately.
Step 7: Ask the person to close the eyes without squeezing them. Press on the inner part of the eye, where the eye meets the nose, for 30 sec.

Step 8: Wipe off excess with a tissue.
Step 9: If more than one drop has been prescribed, wait for 3–4 min before giving the second drop.
Step 10: If another eye drop medication has been prescribed, wait for 5–15 min before giving the second medication.
Step 11: Wash your hands.

Administration of Eye Ointment/Eye Gel

Step 1: Wash your hands with soap and water then dry them.
Step 2: Tilt the older person's head back.
Step 3: Uncap the tube of eye ointment or gel.
Step 4: Pull the lower lid away from the eye using the index finger.
Step 5: Squeeze a ribbon of the ointment or gel into the pocket of the lower eye lid. Do not touch the tip against the eyelid or anything else.
Step 6: Clean the tip of the tube with a clean tissue. Replace the cap immediately.
Step 7: Ask the person to close the eyes without squeezing them for 1–2 min.
Step 8: Wipe off excess with a tissue.
Step 9: Wash your hands.

Performance Skill #31c: Administration of Ear Drops

Step 1: Wash your hands and dry them thoroughly.
Step 2: Shake the bottle gently.
Step 3: Put the bottle on a solid surface and remove the dropper carefully. Make sure that the dropper does not touch any surface.
Step 4: Ask the person to lie on the side with the infected ear facing upwards.
Step 5: Give the required number of drops.
Step 6: Put the dropper back into the bottle and tighten the cap.
Step 7: The person remains in the position for 5 min. Any excess of the ear drops can be wiped away after that.

Performance Skill #32: Administration of Medications via a Nasogastric Tube (NGT)

Step 1: Prepare the medicine.

Tablet (including sugar-coated and film-coated ones):
- Crush the tablet using a tablet crusher or a mortar and pestle.
- Alternatively, dissolve the tablet in a syringe barrel of water.

Capsule:
- Open the capsule and dissolve the powder in water.
- If it is a soft gelatin capsule it can be dissolved in water too, but you should remove any bits of gelatine that are not dissolved.

Liquid medicine:
- Depending on the osmolarity, some of the medicines may be acceptable in their own form, and some thicker ones are to be diluted with 10–30 mL of water.

Step 2: If the medication must be taken on an empty stomach, the milk feed must not be given half an hour before giving the medication and you should only start giving the milk feed an hour after giving the medication.

Step 3: Give the medication via an NGT with a syringe. If a second liquid medication is to be given, flush with 5–10 mL of water between the two medications.

Step 4: Flush with 30 mL of water after the last medication.

Note

Medications that are not suitable to be administer via an NGT included:

- Extended-release, sustained-release or enteric-coated tablets;
- Tablets to be taken under the tongue.

Special considerations:

Medications	What to do
Phenytoin	Stop the milk feed 2 hrs before giving phenytoin and resume the milk feed 2 hrs after. Flush the tube with 60 mL of water after giving phenytoin.
Carbamazepine suspension	Mix with an equal amount of water before giving the medication.
Warfarin	Stop the milk feed 1 hr before and after giving the medication.
Ciprofloxacin, levofloxacin	Crush the tablet thoroughly and mix it with 20–60 mL of water. Stop the milk feed 1 hr before giving the mediciation and 2 hrs after.

Performance Skill #33: Special Diets

Special Diets

- *Diet for an older person with high cholesterol*

Recommended Food	Food to be Avoided
• Oatmeal, oat bran, high-fibre food (especially soluble fibre) • Fish and omega-3 fatty acids • Walnuts, almonds and other nuts • Fresh fruit • Plant sterols	• Saturated fat in fatty meats, poultry skin, full-fat dairy products, coconut oil, palm oil, lard • Trans fat in hard margarine, shortening and some processed foods • Alcohol

- *Diet for an older person with diabetes*

The glycaemic index (GI): measures how a carbohydrate-containing food raises blood glucose. Foods are ranked based on how they compare to a reference food — either glucose or white bread.

Low-GI Food (Less Than 55)	Medium-GI Food (56–69)	High-GI Food (70 or More)
• Oatmeal, oat bran, muesli • Sweet potato, corn, yam, peas, lentils • Most fruits, non-starchy vegetables and carrots	• Whole wheat, rye, pita bread • Quick oats • Brown rice, basmati rice, couscous	• White bread, bagel • Cornflakes, instant oats • White rice • Russet potato, pumpkin • Pretzels, pop corn • Melons, pineapple

A diabetic older person should avoid food with a high GI and choose food with a low GI. However, the total amount of low-GI food is also important. If a large amount of low-GI food is consumed, the blood sugar may be high too.

- *Diet for an older person with hypertension*
  Reduce sodium in the diet:

— Change to a table salt which is low in sodium, e.g. PANSALT®.
— Eat fewer processed foods which have a high salt content, e.g. potato chips and bacon.
— Read food labels — If possible, choose low-sodium alternatives to the food and beverages that you usually buy.

- *Diet for an older person with gout*
  Foods high in purine to avoid if possible or to avoid during flare-ups:

— All internal organs of animals and birds — liver, kidney, brain, pancreas;
— Rich game — venison, gamebird pigeon, black chicken;
— Meat extracts — gravy, chicken essence, *bak kut teh*;
— Certain fishes/shellfish — salmon, herring, mackerel, anchovy, sardine, cockle, mussel, scallop, prawn;
— Certain vegetables — spinach, peas, beans, peanuts, carrot;
— Products of beans — bean curd, soya bean drink, bean sprouts, bean cake, mooncake, legumes;
— Fruits — strawberries, strawberry jam, durian, tomato, tomato sauce;
— Alcohol — beer, champagne, brandy, whisky, port.

- *Diet for an older person on warfarin*

There is no need to change or restrict the food, but an older person should eat about the same amount of foods which are high or low in vitamin K each week.

Foods High in Vitamin K		Foods Low in Vitamin K	
Asparagus	Lettuce	Apple	Fish
Green beans	Mungo beans	Banana	Lamb
Blackberries	Mustard greens	Beef	Lemon
Blueberries	Peas	All cereals	Melon
Broccoli	Pine nuts	(including	Orange
Brussel sprouts	Raisins	flour, etc.)	Peach
Cabbage	Sugar snap peas	Cherries	Pork
Chicory	Soybeans	Chicken	Shellfish
Collard greens	Spinach	Cranberries	Strawberries
Cranberry juice	Swiss chard		Tofu (bean curd)
Kale	Watercress		
Kiwi fruit			

Supplements

Note that supplements may interact with some medicines that the older person is taking or may worsen his or her condition. Check with the doctor or pharmacist if starting a new supplement for the person. Do not assume that if the supplement is from a natural source it is safe. Supplements, whether from natural or synthetic sources, can be unsafe.

Supplement	Not Suitable for Older Persons in the Following Circumstances
Glucosamine	• Allergic to seafood; to choose a vegetarian glucosamine option • May increase blood sugar; to monitor the diabetic older person's blood sugar level
Ginkgo biloba	• On blood-thinning medications as Ginkgo biloba thins the blood • With diabetes; need to monitor the blood glucose level • With a history of seizures • On certain medications, e.g. fluoxetine, medicines changed by the liver (cytochrome P450)

Panax ginseng	• On blood-thinning medications, as Panax ginseng interferes with blood clotting • With diabetes, as Panax ginseng may lower the blood glucose level • With autoimmune disease, e.g. systemic lupus erythematosus (SLE), rheumatoid arthritis (RA), multiple sclerosis • With a hormone-sensitive condition, e.g. breast cancer, uterine cancer, ovarian cancer, endometriosis, uterine fibroids • With insomnia • With schizophrenia • On medications changed by the liver (cytochrome P450)
Evening primrose oil	• With bleeding disorders • With epilepsy or seizures • With schizophrenia • Scheduled for surgery; to stop EPO at least 2 wk before surgery
Fish oil	• With bleeding disorders • With bipolar disorder or depression • Fish oil in high doses may make blood sugar control difficult; to monitor when taking it • With an implanted defibrillator

MODULE 4: EQUIPMENT MANAGEMENT

Performance Skill #34: Using a Hospital Bed

(1) *Manual hand crank bed*

The cranks is usually located at the foot of the bed. If must be turned manually to change the height or position of the bed.

(2) *Electric bed*

This has a motor and is plugged into electricity. It has a control pad which looks like a remote control, for changing the height or position of the bed.

Performance Skill #35: Using a Pressure-Relieving Air Mattress

Step 1: Secure the air mattress to the normal mattress.
Step 2: Place the air pump in the appropriate location; some models may be secured to the foot of the bed.
Step 3: Plug in the electrical supply and on the unit.
Step 4: Choose a suitable setting (usually according to the weight of the older person).

Note

It is better to get the 4-inch-thick mattress than the 2-inch-thick one for a totally dependent or vegetative older person.

Performance Skill #36: Using a Bedpan or Commode

Using a Bedpan

Step 1: Explain the procedure to the older person.
Step 2: Put on gloves.
Step 3: Lower the headrest of the bed and have the person lie on his or her back.
Step 4: Assist the person to roll onto his or her side away from you.
Step 5: Place a waterproof, absorbent pad below the person's buttock.
Step 6: Gently slide the bedpan under the person. Hold it and slowly roll the person back onto his or her back and up onto the bedpan.

Step 7: Raise the headrest if possible, as it is easier for the person to pass urine or motion in a sitting position.
Step 8: Allow the person some privacy.
Step 9: Lower the headrest when the person is done.
Step 10: While holding onto the bedpan, roll the person gently onto his or her side and slide out the bedpan.
Step 11: Clean the person's genitals and buttocks. Pass him or her a wet tissue to clean the hands.
Step 12: Measure and record the output. Empty the bedpan and clean it.
Step 13: Remove the gloves and wash your hands.

Using a Commode

Step 1: Put the commode chair against the wall if possible or lock the wheels.
Step 2: Check that the bucket is in place.
Step 3: Transfer the older person to the commode chair.
Step 4: Let the person have some privacy.
Step 5: Put on a pair of gloves.
Step 6: Help the person to clean up and transfer him or her back to bed.
Step 7: Measure and record the output. Empty the bucket and clean it.
Step 8: Remove the gloves and wash your hands.

Performance Skill #37: Using an Oxygen Concentrator, an Intranasal Cannula or a Mask

Using an Oxygen Concentrator

Step 1: Plug the oxygen concentrator into the electrical outlet.
Step 2: Power on the concentrator and let it start up.
Step 3: When the concentrator is on, there will be a floating black ball visual inside the flow meter. This should be adjusted with the knob and set at the prescribed flow rate.
Step 4: Connect the cannula or mask to the oxygen concentrator and place it on the older person.

Using an Intranasal Cannula

Step 1: Connect the intranasal cannula to the oxygen concentrator.
Step 2: Insert one prong into each nostril.
Step 3: Loop the cannula around the ears.

Using a Mask*

Step 1: Connect the mask to the oxygen concentrator.
Step 2: Place the mask over the older person's nose and mouth. Secure the strap behind his or her head.

*This can give a higher concentration of oxygen compared to using a cannula.

Performance Skill #38: Using an AeroChamber®

AeroChamber with Mask

Step 1: Remove the cap of the inhaler. Shake the inhaler.
Step 2: Insert the inhaler to the back of the chamber.
Step 3: Put the mask on the face and ensure an effective seal for the nose and mouth.
Step 4: Ask the older person to slowly breathe in, then press the inhaler.
Step 5: Maintain the seal for 5–6 breaths, then remove the mask.

AeroChamber with Mouthpiece

Step 1: Remove the cap of the inhaler. Shake the inhaler.
Step 2: Insert the inhaler to the back of the chamber.
Step 3: Place the mouthpiece in the older person's mouth, and ensure that the mouthpiece is sealed with the person's mouth.
Step 4: Ask the person to slowly breathe in, then press the inhaler.
Step 5: Maintain the position for 5–6 breaths with the person breathing slowly, then remove the Aerochamber from his or her mouth.

Performance Skill #39: Using a Nebuliser Machine

Step 1: Wash your hands and ensure that the nebuliser is clean.

Step 2: Pour the prescribed amount of medications into the nebuliser cup. Do note that sometimes saline needs to be added to the nebuliser cup.
Step 3: Connect the nebuliser cup to the nebulising machine via the tubing.
Step 4: Attach the mouthpiece or mask to the nebuliser cup and switch on the machine.
Step 5: If using a mouthpiece, put it into the mouth of the older person. He or she is to breathe in and out slowly through the mouth, until all the medicine is gone. If using a mask, place it over the person's face and he or she is to breathe in and out slowly.
Step 6: The treatment should take about 10 min, till all the medicine is gone. Remove the mouthpiece or mask from the person and clean the nebuliser cup.

Performance Skill #40: Changing and Cleaning the Inner Tube of Non-ventilated Tracheotomised Older Persons

Step 1: Wash your hands and put on gloves.
Step 2: Temporarily disconnect any oxygen delivery device via a trachy mask, if any.
Step 3: Unlock the tracheostomy inner tube.
Step 4: Remove the inner tube and soak it in water with bicarbonate powder added.
Step 5: Insert the replacement tube and lock it into place. Put back the trachy mask, if any.
Step 6: Assess the older person's breathing and check the patency of the airway. Changing the tube may stimulate coughing, and suctioning may be required.
Step 7: The inner tube should be cleaned with sterile, warm water and left to air-dry.

Performance Skill #41: Using a Suction Machine and Suction Catheters

Step 1: Wash your hands with soap and water, then dry them thoroughly. Put on sterile plastic gloves.
Step 2: Connect one end of the 4-inch tubing to the suction port of the collection container, and the other end to the suction catheter.

Step 3: Check that all the tubes are secured. Turn the suction machine on. Adjust the pressure to the desired level. Start from 60 mmHg, and slowly increase it to 120 mmHg if required.

Step 4: Place the older person in a comfortable position, with the head supported by a pillow.

Step 5: Place the suction catheter into the person's mouth or tracheostomy tube and ease it towards the back of the throat or into the tracheostomy tube. The suction catheter should only be near to the back of the throat. If the person starts to gag, remove the catheter immediately.

Step 6: Suction 10 sec at a time, moving in a circular motion. Suction some distilled water into the catheter between suctions. It is recommended to repeat not more than three times per session, with a 20–30 sec break in between.

Step 7: Turn off the suction machine when you are done.

Step 8: Disconnect the suction catheter from the tubing.

Step 9: Rinse the suction catheter and disinfect it. Change it daily if possible and when it is visibly soiled.

Performance Skill #42: Using a Hydraulic Lift for Transfers

Sling lifts or sit-to-stand lifts for transferring older persons are available commercially. However, owing to space restrictions on HDB flats, they are not commonly used.

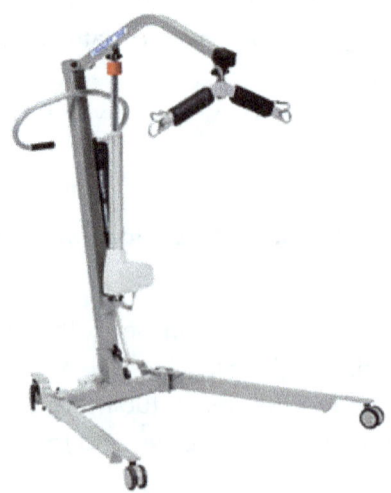

MODULE 5: HOME ENVIRONMENT ASSESSMENT, REHABILITATION AND INFECTION CONTROL

Performance Skill #43: Decluttering and Lighting the Home for an Older Person

Step 1: Make a home environment assessment to look for potential areas that may cause an elderly person to trip and fall. Allow a wide and easily accessible path wherever possible. Remove any clutter as much as possible.

Step 2: Check for proper lighting at night, especially in the bedroom and toilet.

Performance Skill #44: Passive Physiotherapy for Prevention of Contractures

Daily passive physiotherapy to move the joints should be done 2–3 times daily, to prevent joint contractures over the elbows, knees and ankles.

Joints to be passively flexed and extended include:

(1) Shoulder joint — gently rotate it, holding the arm firmly.
(2) Elbow joint — flex, extend, supinate and pronate the elbow with one hand above and one below the joint.
(3) Wrist joint — gently rotate it, holding the hand firmly.
(4) Multiple joints of the hand — open and close the hand, gently flexing and extending the fingers.
(5) Hip and knee joints — lift the leg up and bend the knee to flex both the hip and knee joints, laterally flex the hip joint slightly and gently as well, if possible.
(6) Ankle joint — extend and flex it gently.

Performance Skill #45: Chest Physiotherapy

Chest physiotherapy is very important for a bed-bound older person with poor expansion of his or her lungs from prolonged bed rest.

Chest physiotherapy should be done before feeding the person to avoid inducing vomiting, and should ideally be done before each feed.

Step 1: The person is to be turned to his or her side, supported by a pillow underneath the body or sitting up and leaning forwards towards the caregiver.
Step 2: The caregiver to cup both hands and percuss over the upper and lower scapular areas. Percussion should last for about 5–10 min for each side.
Step 3: During the percussion, monitor and remove any secretions or mucus being expectorated and clean them off the oral cavity.

Performance Skill #46: Use of Personal Protective Equipment (PPE)

Recognising Various PPEs

(1) *Latex or vinyl gloves*
   (a) Use non-powdered gloves if allergic to powdered ones.
   (b) They come in S, M, L sizes.
(2) *3-ply mask*
   (a) This is available in a child or adult size, some with loops or tie strings.
   (b) How to put on the mask:
      (i) Wash your hands and dry them thoroughly.
      (ii) Unfold the pleats, making sure that they are facing down.
      (iii) Place the mask over the nose, mouth and chin.
      (iv) Fit the flexible nose piece over the bridge of the nose. Press it down to fit the bridge.
      (v) Secure the mask with the tie strings (the upper string is to be tied on top of the head above the ears, and the lower string at the back of the neck), or with the loop behind the ears on both sides.
      (vi) Ensure that there are no gaps on either side of the mask, and adjust it to fit.
      (vii) Do not let the mask hang from the neck.
      (viii) To remove the mask untie the tie string below and then the tie string above, and handle the mask using the upper string.

(3) *N95 mask*
    (a) N95 masks are available in different models to fit faces of varying sizes.
    (b) How to put on and take off the mask:
        (i) Wash your hands and them dry thoroughly.
        (ii) Position the mask in your hands with the nose piece at your fingertips.
        (iii) Cup the mask in your hand, allowing the head bands to hang below your hand. Hold the mask under your chin, with the nose piece up.
        (iv) The top strap (on single or double strap respirators) goes over and rests at the top back of your head. The bottom strap is positioned around the neck and below the ears. Do not criss-cross the straps.
        (v) Place the fingertips of both your hands at the top of the metal nose clip (if present). Slide the fingertips down both sides of the metal strip to mould the nose area to the shape of your nose.
        (vi) Remove the mask by pulling the bottom strap over the back of the head, followed by the top strap, without touching the front of the mask.
(4) *Gown*
    Sterile gowns are available but are infrequently used in the home setting.

MODULE 6: BASIC WOUND MANAGEMENT AND DRESSING

Performance Skill #46: Care of Superficial Wounds

Step 1: Wash your hands and dry them thoroughly. Prepare the dressing set and the various types of dressings needed.

Step 2: Clean the wound with water or normal saline as required. Clean it from the middle outwards, using cotton/gauze and forceps.

Step 3: Apply antibiotic ointment or powder as instructed.

Step 4: Use the primary dressing as instructed — Melolin dressing, hydro-colloid foam dressings of various brands, etc.

Step 5: Use the secondary dressing as instructed — usually a waterproof film dressing like Tegaderm®.

Performance Skill #47: Care for Wounds with Cavitation

Step 1: Wash your hands and dry them thoroughly. Prepare the dressing set and the various types of dressings needed.

Step 2: Clean the wound with water or normal saline as required. Clean it from the middle outwards, using cotton/gauze and forceps.

Step 3: Apply antibiotic powder or gel (a hydrocolloid gel such as Duoderm®) as instructed.

Step 4: Use the primary dressing as instructed — a calcium alginate dressing such as Algisite M® for exudative wounds or simple gauze for packing the cavity.

Step 5: Use the secondary dressing as instructed — usually a more absorbent dressing, such as Gamgee®.

Step 6: Use the tertiary protective waterproof film dressing, such as Tegaderm®.

Performance Skill #48: Recognising Bedsores

Step 1: Recognise highly pressurised areas such as the sacral area, heels, elbows and even the pinna.

Step 2: Recognise the development of a bedsore: the pressurised area turning red, changes in hardness, warm to the touch. The red discolouration does not return to the normal skin colour even after removal of any pressure. This can be considered a stage 1 pressure sore.

Step 3: Recognise more advanced sores, such as skin breakdown, sore infection and cavitation. These are stage 2–4 pressure sores.

Performance Skill #49: Recognising Infected Sores and Wounds

Step 1: The skin around the sore turns red.
Step 2: Swelling can be observed and there may be pus from the wound.
Step 3: The older person complains of pain over the area.
Step 4: The person develops fever or delirium.
Step 5: Refer the person to health professionals (doctors or nurses) for evaluation.

Performance Skill #50: Understanding and Recognising Products Used in Wound Care

Products Commonly Used in Singapore

Sterile basic dressing set   • Contains items that are commonly needed when doing wound cleaning/dressing   • Usually contains sterile cotton balls, sterile gauze, disposable forceps, patient drapes, hand towel and limpet bag
Gauze   • Sterile or non-sterile   • Can be used as primary or secondary dressing   • Highly permeable   • May stick to wound, making it difficult to remove
Low-adherent dressing pad   • Can absorb small amount of exudate   • Can be applied directly to wound and will not stick to it   • Easier to remove when changing dressing

Alginate dressing • Made from brown seaweed • Absorbs exudate to form gel in wound • For moderately to severely exudating wound • Requires secondary dressing, usually gauze • Available as sheet or rope	
Hydrogel dressing • For dry or minimally exudating wound • Donates moisture to wound to help break down dry dead tissue • Requires secondary dressing	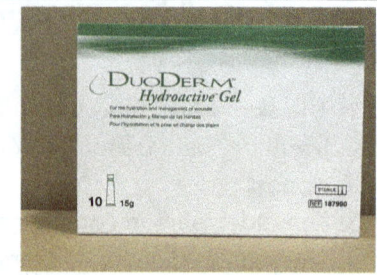
Adhesive hydrocolliod dressing • Contains gelatin, pectin or cellulose bonded to carrier of semi-permeable film or foam sheet • Absorbs exudate slowly to form gel-like mass • Gel-like mass may be foul-smelling • For minimally to moderately exudating wound • Waterproof and impermeable to air and bacteria	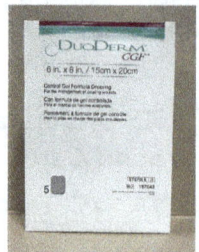 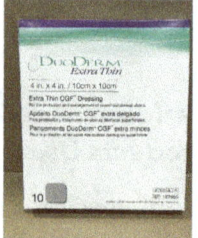
Foam dressing • For moderately to severely exudating wound • Protects and cushions wound • Some products have adhesive border, others do not. If adhesive border is not present, tape may be used to secure dressing	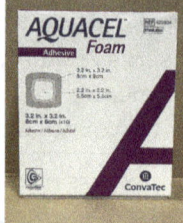

Antimicrobial dressing • Typically contains either silver or iodine	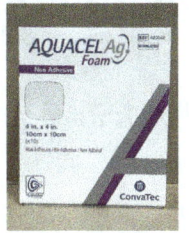 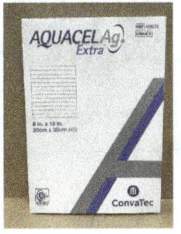
Semi-permeable film • Waterproof dressing to promote moist environment • Allows visual checks • Used as secondary dressing	

Note: The products shown are examples and not an exhaustive list: The photos are from ConvaTec.

MODULE 7: RECOGNITION OF EMERGENT CONDITIONS

Performance Skill #51: Recognising Delirium in an Older Person

Delirium can manifest as either agitation, aggression or depressed, hypoactive behaviours. A trained caregiver by the side of the older person daily will be the best judge of delirium for him or her. Changes from daily behaviour such as vocal disruptions, resisting care, or aggressive, attacking tendencies or verbalisation of visual or auditory hallucinations, i.e. seeing small children running about, dead relatives visiting or strangers breaking into the house, setting fire, etc., are the more easily recognised forms of delirium. Hypoactive symptoms, such as lethargy, drowsiness, general physical decline and weakness, are less noticeable at times and help may be unsought or delayed. Many factors from constipation, pain, life-threatening infections or heart attacks can first manifest as delirium in a dependent older person.

The caregiver is to recognise and flag such observations, and refer the person to health a professional (doctor or nurse) timely for further evaluation.

Performance Skill #52: Recognising Dyspnoea

Step 1: Recognise the verbal complaint of breathlessness in an older person if he or she is still able to communicate.
Step 2: Monitor the respiratory rate. A rate of more than 30 breaths a minute may signify an underlying problem of oxygenation and ventilation.
Step 3: Look for discolouration of the lips and nail beds (turning purplish or blue) which indicates cyanosis. Check for desaturation if a pulse oximeter is available.
Step 4: Refer the person to a health professional (doctor or nurse) for further evaluation.

Performance Skill #53: Recognising Oedema, Localised or Generalised

Step 1: Recognise swelling over the periorbital area, face, trunk and limbs.

Step 2: Do measurements of the body part if possible, for charting the size of the progressive swelling.
Step 3: Refer the older person to a health professional (doctor or nurse) for further evaluation.

Performance Skill #54: Recognising Chest Infection

Step 1: Monitor for fever.
Step 2: Recognise chest infection symptoms.
- Cough, either productive or non-productive
- Colour of sputum and any blood stain

Step 3: Recognise any onset of vomiting or delirium in the older person.
Step 4: If the respiratory rate is more than 30 breaths a minute, seek prompt evaluation and treatment.
Step 5: Refer the person to a health professional (doctor or nurse) for further evaluation.

Performance Skill #55: Recognising Urinary Tract Infection

Step 1: Monitor for fever.
Step 2: Recognise urinary infection symptoms.
- Foul smelling urine — very different from the usual smell on diaper-changing
- Note any pus or blood-stained urine on the diapers

Step 3: Recognise urinary retention.
- Diapers not wet after 6–8 hr
- Palpable or visible hard lump over the lower abdomen, just on top of the pelvic bone

Step 4: Recognise any onset of vomiting or delirium in the older person.
Step 5: Refer the person to a health professional (doctor or nurse) for further evaluation.

Performance Skill #56: Recognising Constipation and Associated Complications

Step 1: Recognise the normal bowel habits of the dependent older person and do bowel-charting.

An example of a bowel chart:

Date	Time	Amount	Remarks
02/01/18	Morning, 7 a.m. – 3 p.m.	Nil	
	Afternoon, 3 p.m. – 11 p.m.	Small amount	Watery
	Night, 11 p.m. – 7 a.m.	Large amount	

Step 2: Recognise the normal stool colour, volume and consistency for the person and take note if that is different from usual.

Step 3: Give regular oral laxatives, a bisacodyl suppository or a fleet enema as instructed by the health professional.

   Inserting a Suppository:

 (i) Lay the person to one side with both knees bent.
 (ii) Pull up the gluteal muscles on the top and ask the person to relax.
 (iii) Lubricate the suppository with an aqueous gel lubricant.
 (iv) Apply light but constant digital pressure over the anal verge to relax the anal muscle.
 (v) Insert the suppository using index finger and gently press the tablet against the rectal wall.

Step 4: Recognise abdominal distension and regurgitation or vomiting as possible signs of constipation.

Step 5: Recognise urinary retention as a possible sign of constipation.

Step 6: Learn and do manual evacuation from the health professional if required.

3 Effects of Aging and Common Diseases

PART 1: EFFECTS OF AGING

Cardiovascular System

Blood vessels become stiffer from loss of elastic fibres, and with that resistance to the flow of blood, and hence the blood pressure, may increase. The hardening of heart valves can also lead to dysfunction of the heart in terms of muscular action and rhythm. In addition, the heart shows a gradual reduction in performance, with a lesser amount of blood pumped out per unit time.

Dentition

Many older persons are usually without a full dentition. The cause is multifactorial, such as long-standing dental caries, periodontal diseases and degenerative factors resulting in loss of dentine, cement and gingiva. A loose tooth may be a concern, especially for persons who have a swallowing impairment, with the risk of aspirating the tooth if it is detached.

Endocrine System

In healthy older persons, the endocrine system should remain unchanged in a disease-free state.

Gastrointestinal System

The gastrointestinal system should not change much apart from a mild decrease in gastric emptying. However, constipation may be more common in the elderly, possibly owing to side effects of chronic medications and immobility.

Haematological System

The bone marrow may have an increase in the adipose tissue content but generally the red and white blood cell content should be comparable to normal ranges.

Musculoskeletal System

There may be a gradual loss of calcium from the bones in older persons, coupled with loss of elasticity of the joints from calcification of the ligaments and tendons. Muscle fibres may atrophy with immobility and inactivity. Regular exercise to maintain muscular strength and flexibility of the joints should always be encouraged. Poor muscular strength may result in poor balancing and thus falls. Falls may result in fractures of osteoporotic bones if both bone health and muscle strength are not maintained.

Renal System

The blood flow to the kidneys is known to be decreased in very old persons, resulting in decreased ability to conserve salt and water. This makes the older person less able to maintain a balance of fluids in the body during disease states and more prone to be either dehydrated or overloaded with fluids. The urinary bladder may also have an increased post-void volume and more uninhibited contractions, making urinary incontinence more frequent in the person. With some decline or changes in diurnal anti-diuretic hormone secretions, the person may need to pass urine at night owing to the continual urine production.

Respiratory System

The stiffening of costal cartilages from calcifications coupled with a certain extent of kyphosis may increase the work of breathing. Otherwise, there should not be any changes in overall airway resistance. The number of alveoli may decrease from fibrosis or atrophy, possibly resulting in a less effective oxygen transfer to the blood.

Sensory System

Vision, hearing and taste all undergo aging processes and may not be as sharp in older persons compared to when they were younger. Taste affects appetite, and hence the risk of malnutrition may be higher with less food intake in older persons. Decline in vision and hearing may cause much anxiety and inconvenience to them.

Skin

Owing to loss of elastic fibres, or a decrease in the collagen content and subcutaneous tissue, the skin loses its elasticity. If that is coupled with thickening of the epidermis and shrinking of the dermis layer, the skin is more prone to shearing forces and tearing. There is a loss of sebaceous glands, with less production of sebum, and the skin gets dehydrated more easily. In addition, there is an increase in vascular malformations resulting in skin tags and senile purpura.

Weight and Height

There is a fat redistribution in the body, with fat around the face getting atrophied. Loss of height from occult vertebral fractures results in kyphosis. Loss of weight of more than 5–10% over a six-month period is cause for concern and should be investigated if intake has been normal.

PART 2: COMMON DISEASES ENCOUNTERED BY CAREGIVERS

Communicable Diseases

Chest Infection

Many of our dependent older persons are partially or fully bed-bound, and on nasogastric tube feeding. They are at high risk for developing chest infections from aspiration pneumonia or getting secondary bacterial infections of the chest from normal flu viral infection or due to poor lung expansion and mucus plugging in the respiratory system.

It is important to constantly monitor for chest infections in a bed-bound older person and do daily chest physiotherapy routines before feeding him or her. For a certain group of older persons with lung pathologies, more invasive management, such as routine suctioning, may be required. This is especially true for older persons who were admitted into intensive care units and had a tracheostomy done for ventilation and suctioning.

When a chest infection is suspected, prompt antibiotic treatment should be started. Chest physiotherapy should be intensified and other supportive pharmacologic treatments, like mucolytic agents or beta 2 adrenergic receptor blocker inhalers, can be started. Caregivers should refer these cases to the health professional if they suspect that there is a chest infection.

Pulmonary Tuberculosis

Pulmonary tuberculosis is a microbial infection which can affect the lungs and other parts of the body. The usual symptoms affecting the lungs are cough with productive sputum which is sometimes blood-stained. The systemic signs are fever, chills, cold sweats and weight loss.

This disease can recur in the body after years of being inactive. It infects the person when he or she is immunocompromised by malnutrition or recurrent infections and hospitalisations.

Urinary Tract Infection

Many older persons are more prone to be constipated owing to medication use and immobility. When an older person is constipated, there is a tendency to develop urinary retention and consequently a urinary tract infection. If left untreated, urinary tract infections may worsen, resulting in life-threatening kidney infections and infections of the blood known as septicaemia.

It is crucial for the caregiver to monitor the urine for its volume and smell, and whether there is pus or blood in the urine. Systemic signs like fever, delirium and vomiting are common as well. Prompt treatment of urinary tract infections can prevent further complications and hospitalisation. Caregiver should refer the older person to health professionals for prompt treatment if they suspect that he or she has a urinary tract infection.

Skin Infection

Owing to a decrease in the dermis layer and subcutaneous layer from aging, the skin may tend to tear more easily. Without the skin covering as a protective layer against microbial agents, skin infections can develop more frequently, especially in a bed-bound individual. Skin infections around pressure sores and ulcers are common as well, and if not treated, they are likely to worsen and cause a systemic infection. Usually, skin infections can be treated successfully with penicillin-based antibiotics. Caregivers should refer the older person to health professionals for prompt treatment if they suspect that he or she has a skin infection.

Herpes Zoster Infection

A herpes zoster infection is caused by a virus known as the varicella-zoster virus (VZV) and manifests as painful skin vesicular lesions, which follow a nerve that supplies a segment of the skin. It occurs in those who are immnunocompromised. It causes severe pain and discomfort, and disseminated zoster infections, if left untreated, can be life-threatening. The caregiver should alert the doctor to start antiviral agents, which are usually very effective in treating the infection. The lesions will generally dry up and drop off, leaving some hypo-pigmented scars at times. Without prompt and proper treatment and pain relief, some older persons can develop "phantom pain" over the affected areas, even when the lesion subsides. Rarely, the infection can cause chronic pain, depression and general decline of the older person.

Non-Communicable Diseases

Palliative Care

Palliative care means keeping the older person comfortable and free of distressing symptoms such as pain, breathlessness and itch. There are dedicated palliative care teams that offer institutional or home-based services. The older persons will most often be on some form of pain relief therapy, like morphine syrup, fentanyl patches or even continuous subcutaneous morphine infusion. Caregivers must follow the instructions of the palliative teams when dealing with an older person on palliative support. They should also know about the types of support available in the community if the person is to be managed at home, such as signing up of certification of the cause of death.

Organ Failure

Heart Failure

Our heart is a vital organ for pumping our blood throughout our body to bring oxygen and nutrients to all the body cells. It has four chambers and two main circulations, serving either the lungs or the rest of the body. For ease of explanation, we will consider a more generalised heart failure. The older person is usually very tired, having breathing difficulties at times owing to accumulation of fluids in the lungs, and may present lower limb oedema (swelling) or even ascites (water accumulating in the abdominal cavity). The symptoms may worsen with any exertion. The person is most likely on multiple medications and sometimes on oxygen therapy. He or she is on strict fluid restrictions and the caregiver may be tasked with monitoring his or her weight daily.

Respiratory Failure

Our lungs have two major functions: to oxygenate and to ventilate. As with heart failure, older persons with lung failure are often breathless on exertion and are usually on long-term oxygen therapy at home. They are very prone to chest infections as well and will need to be monitored for symptoms like increased frequency of productive cough, chest pain, fever, lethargy and even delirium. Many such older persons are on inhalers and even nebulisers at home. Caregivers will need to have proper knowledge and skills to administer these therapies at home.

Renal Failure

Our kidneys serve to produce urine and excrete any waste from the bloodstream. They are very important for stimulating blood production and maintaining a balance of the electrolytes, and have an effect on the calcium level.

Older persons with renal failure are usually on dialysis, using either blood or the peritoneal (abdomen) cavity. However, there are very frail older persons who may not be suitable for or refuse such renal therapies. They are on multiple medications, especially certain medications to help them produce urine for excretion. They are very prone to swelling, breathlessness and generalised itch. Medications to treat the complications of kidney failure are usually on standby at home and the caregivers are taught when and how to use them. As with older persons with heart failure, older persons with renal failure are on strict fluid restrictions and should undergo daily monitoring of weight and swelling of the feet.

Liver Failure

Older persons with liver cirrhosis can be very fragile and very sick within a very short duration. They are very prone to delirium from encephalopathy, and the more terminal ones are very prone to recurrent seizures. It is very important to take note of any constipation, as any degree of constipation can result in delirium and will entail intensive medical support in hospital. The person can have very generalised swelling, especially ascites. Symptoms may be very difficult to resolve despite draining and tapping the fluids.

The older persons are also usually on multiple medications, and high doses of lactulose to prevent constipation.

Chronic Diseases

Diabetes Mellitus

Diabetes mellitus is a common chronic disease in Singapore. It is a systemic disease characterised by high blood glucose. The therapies for diabetes mellitus include diet control, oral medications and even subcutaneous injections of insulin. Monitoring for low blood glucose is at times more crucial than higher readings. It will be good for the caregivers to learn to use the blood glucometer to monitor the fasting and 2 hr post meal readings for older persons on oral medications. This will be required if the person is on insulin injections for the disease. A range of 5–15 is acceptable and an

Hba1c value of less than 8.5% may be acceptable for a totally dependent and non-communicative older person.

Hypertension

Hypertension is one of the most common chronic diseases in Singapore. It is characterised by a blood pressure reading of more than 140 mmHg systolic and 90 mmHg diastolic. Many of our bed-bound older persons have quite good control, either with or without oral medications. For older persons who are still ambulatory, it will be good to check the blood pressure before giving the anti-hypertensives. If the systolic blood pressure is less than 100 mmHg, avoid giving further anti-hypertensives, in order to prevent subsequent hypotension and shock. All anti-hypertensives have their own side effects and the caregiver should take note of any changes when the person is being started on a new medication. For example, an ACE inhibitor like lisinopril may cause coughing, and calcium channel blockers like amlodipine may cause foot swelling.

Dyslipidaemia

An increase in the level of cholesterol, especially LDL cholesterol, is a risk factor for heart disease and stroke. Many older persons with a history of heart disease or stroke are put on anti-cholesterol medications. Side effects are rare, but they can cause liver problems and muscle aches. Caregivers are to take note and feed back to the physician if there are signs such as jaundice or if the older person complains of generalised muscle pain. The physician in charge will usually order some lab tests to further evaluate the physical complaints.

Heart Diseases Including Ischaemic Heart Disease and Atrial Fibrillation

Many older persons with ischaemic heart disease are on multiple medications and a standby medication known as glyceryl trinitrate (GTN). GTN is often given as a tablet to be placed under the tongue to relieve chest discomfort. It also comes as a spray to be administered under the tongue as well. For many older persons with irregular heart rhythms, usually resulting in the heart beating much faster, monitoring both the heart rate by feeling the apex beating of the heart and pulse rate will be helpful. Any complaint from the person of feeling the heart beating very fast or irregularly should be treated seriously and he or she should be referred to the doctor for further evaluation.

Gout and Swellings of the Joints and Limbs

Sudden, painful swelling over the joints and limbs may occur during the care of a dependent older person. The most common cause is gout if the older person is still on oral feeding, with a history of gout and after a major festive season. However, some older persons on blood-thinning medications (anti-coagulants like warfarin) can develop bleeding into the joints and muscles. This condition is less painful than gout, but the caregiver must alert the health professional for an urgent review to rule out over-warfarinisation. Rarely, with a combination of osteoporosis, decreased flexibility of the joints from tendon and ligament calcifications, and passive physiotherapy or transferring, fracture can occur in a dependent, bed-bound older person. Although already bed-bound and non-ambulant, the person should still be transferred to a hospital for pain control and blood transfusions if bleeding into the fracture site is significant.

Eye Diseases — Eye Dryness and Cataracts

Eye dryness and Cataracts are common eye complaints in older persons. The symptoms of eye dryness include irritable eyes, itchy eyes and even teary eyes with a yellowing residue at the lower corner of the eyelids. Regular eye lubricants and massaging of the areas around the tear ducts may help.

For cataracts, the persons should be referred for cataract surgeries as much as possible if they are still ambulant and have good cognition.

Hearing Impairment and Earwax

Older persons with hearing impairment should be checked for earwax. Chronic impaction of earwax can cause discomfort and even ear canal infections. Older persons with hearing impairment can also be referred for hearing aids if suitable.

Neurological/Psychological Diseases

Stroke

Older persons with a major stroke constitute a large proportion of home-bound, dependent older persons. Apart from taking medications to lower the risk of further strokes, routine physiotherapy to maintain joint flexibility and prevent contractures is an important aspect of the care as well. For those already bed-bound and on nasogastric tube feeding, prevention of complications must be taken into consideration. Psychological complications of the stroke, such as depression and dementia, should be closely monitored as well. Routine monitoring of vital signs should be done by the caregiver. Symptoms of any infections arising from being bed-bound and possible side effects of the medications should be made known to the caregiver.

Parkinsonism

In the home care setting, we often see older persons with advanced Parkinson's disease, where they are not able to ambulate or are already on nasogastric tube feeding. Apart from doing routine passive physiotherapy to keep the joints flexible, constipation may be a routine issue for such persons. For older persons who are still communicative, titration of Parkinsonism medications is very important. Too high a dose may cause hallucinations and behavioural problems while too low a dose may not treat the stiffness and tremors adequately. For those who can still ambulate, great care is to be taken when they do so, to prevent falls and fractures.

Dementia

Older persons with dementia, especially in the more advanced stage, may be bed-bound and on nasogastric tube feeding, owing to physical and functional decline with poor intake of food. Those in the moderate-to-severe stage are often frail and require supervision or may be partially dependent on the caregiver for all the ADLs. During the early-to-moderate stage, some may exhibit disruptive behavioural issues like aggression and accusative behaviours resulting in caregiver stress and family conflict at times. Both the older persons and the carers may develop depression at this stage.

The caregivers may need respite from constantly taking care and managing the behaviours of the demented older persons over prolonged periods. There are many community support centres which are home based, like iPal or CREST. Other programmes include the Alzheimer's Disease Associations of Singapore–run New Horizon Care Centres and hospital-run programmes such as Charitas.

Epilepsy

Older persons with prior neurological trauma or pathologies such as stroke may be more prone to develop seizures. They are usually already on anti-epileptic medications but may develop breakthrough seizures, especially during an episode of urinary tract infection or even a recurrent stroke. Some caregivers are instructed to start a seizure chart at home to monitor the frequency and duration of any arising seizures. Standby rectal diazepam maybe prescribed. It is a medication used to abort a severe seizure. The caregiver will be taught how to administer the rectal tube if the need arises.

4 Caregiver Stress Management

Caring for a chronically sick older person puts all caregivers at risk of caregiver stress. In the case of caring for a demented older person with behavioural issues, the burnout rate is much higher among these caregivers.

There are various ways to manage caregiver stress. The caregiver should:

- Have proper knowledge of the care situation;
- Know strategies for handling the situation;
- Have a coping mechanism to alleviate caregiver stress;
- Know about respite care services for older persons;

Support for the caregiver is crucial in any successful care planning for a chronically sick older person. Hence, a well-trained caregiver who knows the care situation and is trained to cope with the known challenges is at a lesser risk for burnout. A trained caregiver should also be familiarised with the various forms of community support available and tap on such support. For example, many home care services may provide bathing services for older persons, and this will help to take off some of the physical pressure of doing the bathing alone for the person. Use of proper equipment can also help the caregiver cope better; a good pressure-relieving mattress, for example, will obviate the need for the caregiver to turn the bed-bound person every 2–4 hr, for bedsore prevention. Moreover, there are support groups that caregivers can join to share coping tips on managing older persons. Day care centres for demented or very dependent older persons are also available but, unfortunately, the waiting lists are always very long.

To have a successful caregiving experience, caregivers should be given a clear care plan from the health professionals and a case manager for each case. The case manager can help the caregiver source for support and link the caregiver up with other services. Caregivers should feel supported by the system or institution they are in.

When a caregiver suffers burnout, respite care for the older person should be considered. However, respite care can be very expensive in general. The person can be transferred to a community hospital, a nursing home or even a home-based respite care programme where another caregiver comes to the house for the care of the person.

Every older person's and every family's resources and coping mechanism are very different. Taking into account what the person expects for his or her care and what the family can provide, the health professionals can formulate a long-term care plan. In this plan, they can educate the person and his or her family on what to expect and all the community resources available, as well as the pros and cons of each supporting service and the costs involved. The subsidies that are available will be discussed in the next chapter.

The care plan can also include advance care planning on the type of support or end-of-life care the person would want, such as the use of nasogastric tube feeding or other, more invasive and advanced treatments, like chemotherapy.

Help available:

(1) *Transitional care*
- Lasts about 3–6 mth from the older person's discharge from hospital.
- Doctors and nurses to do home visits to follow up the person after discharge from hospital to manage certain conditions.
- To check with each hospital for availability, cost and referral.

(2) *Interim care*
- Provides a caregiver in blocks of 12 hr each day for 2 wk or 24 hr for 1 wk immediately after discharge from hospital.
- Subsidised service provided by Thye Hua Kwan Ensuite Home Care and other participating charities or social enterprises.
- To check with each hospital or organisation for availability, cost and referral.

(3) *Home care*
- Provides a caregiver to help with showering/bathing, and for companionship, escorting to medical appointments, meal preparation and exercise for a few hours a day.
- Subsidised service available from Thye Hua Kwan Ensuite Home Care and NTUC Eldercare.
- Private service available from Homage, Jaga-Me, Global Active Caregivers, Comfort Keepers and a few others.

(4) *Elder or dementia day care or day rehabilitation service*
- Dependent or non-dependent older persons will stay in these care centres during the day.
- Meals may be provided there.
- Physiotherapy support will be provided in day rehabilitation services.

(5) *Respite care in a nursing home or community hospital*
- Institutionalised care of chronically sick older persons.
- Will usually require a formal referral from the team seeing the person and a recent chest X-ray to clear him or her person of any active pulmonary tuberculosis or chest infection before admission.

HOW TO IDENTIFY CAREGIVER STRESS?

In the author's many talks on caregivers and caregiver stress, one question routinely pops up: How do we identify caregiver stress and caregiver burnout? There are many different surveys and caregiver stress checklists online for identifying caregiver stress, one of which is the Zarit Burden Interview. The interview gives a set of scores which can identify little or no burden to severe burden in the caregiver.

Other features of stress or burnout can be manifested as physical or mental complaints such as:

- Feelings of depression and frustration
- Constant fatigue
- Sudden weight loss or gain
- Insomnia
- Headaches

No two caregiving experiences are alike, but they may be more similar if the caregivers are dealing with the similar clinical scenarios which the seniors suffer from. Always seek help if you are a caregiver undergoing caregiver stress or burnout!

DIFFERENT CAREGIVER STRESS IN DIFFERENT CLINICAL SITUATIONS

Palliative Care

Seniors suffering from terminal diseases such as metastatic cancers or end stage organ failures may be treated for symptoms such as pain or other discomfort. A good proportion of seniors may be admitted into a hospice for end-of-life care, but some seniors and their families choose to stay at home for the terminal care. There are multiple excellent home hospice services which are run by charities or non-governmental organisations funded heavily by the government. Some of these services run 24/7. The main weakness in this situation is often that the caregivers themselves are poorly trained and educated in the caregiving strategies. Palliative care is traditionally seen to be shorter-term care and often the training and support of the caregivers are poorer compared to those with long-term care services. There is less likelihood of the family getting a formal stay-in caregiver and usually the spouse or the children take over the physical and daily care of the older person. And without formal training and directions, some of the caregivers may feel very lost.

It will be good for the family to decide in favour of an informal caregiver and send the caregiver for short caregiving courses first to empower him or her in the care journey.

Seniors with Dementia or a Psychiatric Illness

Caring for an ambulating and physically functional senior with dementia or some other psychiatric illness can be both physically and mentally draining for any caregiver. More than a quarter of caregivers are caring for seniors with varying degrees of cognitive impairment. Caregiving for a person with dementia is associated with high levels of stress caused by associated behavioural disturbances, intense physical needs, and a need for constant vigilance. Burnout and mental breakdowns from caring for such individuals are common, with high a incidence of nursing home care placement as an eventual solution for the family.

The caregiver in this situation will need to understand the disease and its progression, as well as understand and apply both non-pharmacological and pharmacological means of controlling behavioural disruptions. He or she must also have knowledge of the community services available to support the care, such as dementia day care centers, or other dementia care support at home. Self-care and good emotional control of daily frustrations will be crucial in maintaining a balanced and controlled caregiving journey.

Seniors with Stroke Disease

Advancement in modern medicine has allowed more stroke survivors to have less severe disabilities, but sometimes this comes at the price of an increased period of dependence in the years of survival ahead. Many of such caregiver journeys can be prolonged, in terms of decades where care and support are needed. Many of these stroke survivors may require assistance in their activities of daily living and instrumental activities of daily living.

The caregiving journey in these scenarios is more a marathon than a 100-metre dash. Planning of financial resources, respite care plans and monitoring of the chronic disease to prevent further complications are some of the mainstays of the management plan.

There are many stoke support units in the community, and the Stroke Support Station (www.s3.org) is one of such community resources. The caregiver can join a disease-based community effort to get support in the form of social and rehabilitative help.

Seniors with Organ Failures

Seniors can also decline and require caregiving when they suffer from end-organ failures, such as cardiac failures after decades of hypertension. Many of such seniors with organ failures can have multiple exacerbations and flare-ups of the disease and require repeated admissions into hospitals. These repeated admissions cause much stress and anxiety among the caregivers. Many acute hospitals have now set up transitional care services to come to the homes of the seniors to offer support and to manage such flare-ups when possible. Many families face dilemmas in older-person care, since many of these seniors are cognitively intact and seniors are uncomfortable and symptomatic when the exacerbations and flare-ups occur.

Good advance care planning can be discussed with the hospital ACP facilitator in such cases. Seniors' preference of care should be sought and, to all intents and purposes, be followed by the institution and the family.

Transition of Care

Transition of care may cause much anxiety to the caregiver. There are three types of transition of care.

Firstly, transition of care needs, for example from oral feeding to tube feeding, or from an ambulant senior to a bed-bound senior. Many new skills are required for the sudden change, and the caregiver will sometimes be unprepared for the new requirements of the care. This is when caregiver skill training comes into play to support the caregiver.

Secondly, transition of care from home to institution. It may mean the end of physical caring but may be more stressful mentally. There may be a feeling of guilt or a constant commute to the care facility or a constant worry over a sudden call from the nursing home about a worsening of the medical condition. Different caregivers will have different mental issues with regard to such a transition. The transition should be recognised by the family, who should be given support as and when required.

Lastly, transition of the love one's passing. With prolonged caregiving, many caregivers can suffer complex grief and a momentary loss of purpose in life and change of their daily routines. They may be less or more depressed, depending on the support given and their intrinsic ability to cope with the losses. Many cases remained unrecognised and may manifest physical symptoms and poor health. The caregivers themselves should recognise whether they are suffering complex grief and a loss of purpose in life and, if so, seek help immediately.

Tips for Caregivers

The caregiver must understand that proper self-care will be the most important factor in the care recipient's outcome. Hence, without proper self-care, the care journey will head for a less ideal outcome.

There are many new technologies and tools to support the care of a dependent older person, and caregivers should maximise the use of them.

It is always good to seek support and help from community resources and to identify oneself as suffering from caregiver stress and burnout. Caring for a dependent older person is always and will always be a team based effort. The caregiver is the most important member of the team and there should always be a team identified to get constant support from throughout the journey. The team can consist of many healthcare and non-healthcare-related professionals. Here are some examples:

- Eldercare legal team with lawyers for issues of welfare/finance and property power of attorney
- Eldercare financial planner team for insurance schemes, reverse housing mortgages, etc.
- Spiritual support team from temples, churches or mosques
- Social and day-to-day support teams for transportation and logistic support (housekeeping, meals, outings, etc); even neighbours can be a potential resource
- Medical support team comprising a long-term care physician, home care nurses, therapists and social workers

Do get an eldercare team formed up today!

5 Financial Support and Useful Information for Eldercare

PART 1: FINANCIAL SUBSIDIES*

Interim Disability Assistance Programme for the Elderly (IDAPE)

Website: https://www.silverpages.sg/financial-assistance/elderly-and-seniors/Interim%20Disability%20Assistance%20Scheme%20For%20the%20Elderly%20(IDAPE)

The Interim Disability Assistance Programme for the Elderly (IDAPE) is an assistance scheme that was set up in 2002 for the group of seniors who were not eligible for ElderShield at the time because they were too old or had pre-existing disabilities.

A monthly cash payout for a maximum of 72 months is given to Singapore citizens who meet the following criteria:

- Born before 30 September 1932 or between 1 October 1932 and 30 September 1962 (both dates inclusive) but with pre-existing disabilities as at 30 September 2002;
- Household monthly income per person of $2,600 or below or annual value of residence of $13,000 or below for households with no income;
- Severely disabled (i.e. unable to perform at least three out of six ADLs*).

*Activities of daily living — washing/bathing, feeding, toileting, transferring, dressing and mobility.

---

*Note that all the information given about financial subsidies is accurate at the point of writing. To get the latest information, go to the websites of the schemes.

The older persons must apply for means testing first:
https://www.silverpages.sg/sites/silverpagesassets/SilverPages%20Assets/Application%20Forms%20(Financial,%20Care%20Services)/Means-Test%20Declaration%20Form.pdf

When the means test has been approved, application for IDAPE will be done. A panel doctor's assessment is required as part of the application:
https://www.silverpages.sg/sites/silverpagesassets/SilverPages%20Assets/Application%20Forms%20(Financial,%20Care%20Services)/AIC%20Scheme%20Application%20Form.PDF

Per Capita Household Monthly Income	Monthly Payout
$0–$1,800	$250
$1,801–$2,600	$150

ElderShield

Website: https://www.moh.gov.sg/content/moh_web/eldershield/about-eldershield.html#4

ElderShield is an insurance scheme introduced by the Ministry of Health to provide financial help to those who are unable to take care of themselves because of severe disabilities.

The scheme gives a cash payout every month to those who are severely disabled — not able to do three or more of the following ADLs: washing, feeding, dressing, toileting, mobility and transferring.

Basic Eldershield 300	Basic Eldershield 400
Insured before 30.09.2007	Insured on or after 30.09.2007
Monthly benefit of $300	Monthly benefit of $400
Benefit payout period of 60 months	Benefit payout period of 72 months

ÉlderShield is administered by different insurance companies, namely NTUC Income, Great Eastern and Aviva, depending on the older person's plan.

A panel doctor's assessment is required as part of the application.

Enhancements for Active Seniors (EASE)

Website: http://www.hdb.gov.sg/cs/infoweb/residential/living-in-an-hdb-flat/for-our-seniors/ease

EASE provides for the following improvements in flats:

- Slip-resistant treatment for floor tiles of up to two bathrooms/ toilets;
- Eight or ten grab bars for first toilet and within the flat, and six grab bars for the second toilet*;
- Up to five ramps within the flat for negotiating one level difference in the flat and/or at a single-step main entrance*

*Where technically feasible.

	Singapore Citizen Households			
Flat Type	1/2/3 Room	4-Room	5-Room	Executive
Older Person's Pay	$125 (5%)	$187.50 (7.5%)	$250 (10%)	$312.50 (12.5%)
Government Pays	$2,375 (95%)	$2,312.50 (92.5%)	$2,250 (90%)	$2,187.50 (87.5%)

Flat owners can choose any or all of the improvements to be done and pay only for what is done.

The eligibility criteria for EASE (Direct Application) are as follows:

(i) Singapore citizen households must have an elderly member who is 65 years old or above, or
(ii) Singapore citizen households with at least one member aged between 60 and 64 years who requires assistance for one or more of the Activities of daily living ADLs.*

*"Activities of daily living" (ADLs) is a term used in healthcare to refer to daily self-care activities within an individual's place of residence. These activities include washing/bathing, dressing, feeding, toileting, mobility and transferring.

If one is applying via (ii), a functional assessment must be done by a Singapore-registered doctor.

Electronic application:
http://services2.hdb.gov.sg/webapp/BN37AWEASE/BN37PMain.jsp

Senior Mobility and Enabling Fund (SMF)

Website: https://www.silverpages.sg/SMF

Category of subsidy	Where to Apply? (MOH-Funded)	Which Seniors Can Apply?	What Can You Get?
Assistive devices	Restructured hospitals, community hospitals, intermediate-and long-term care (ILTC) service providers, Agency for Integrated Care (AIC)	Those who require a device as tested by a qualified assessor (e.g. therapist, registered nurse, doctor or audiologist)	Up to 90% subsidy of the actual cost of the device. *The subsidy cap will depend on the cost of the type of device needed.*
Transport (via Specialised Vehicles)	Day rehabilitation centres (DRCs)	Community–ambulant on wheelchairs and requiring specialised transport	Amount of subsidy will depend on means testing.
	Dialysis centres	Community–ambulant on wheelchairs and requiring specialised transport	
	Dementia day care centres (DDCCs)	All clients requiring specialised transport	
Home Healthcare Items	Home-based healthcare services (home medical/home nursing)	Must undergo assessment to determine the need and the type of healthcare items required	
	AIC's Singapore Programme for Integrated Care for the Elderly (SPICE)		

Criteria for Assistive Devices

To be eligible, the senior:

- Must be aged 60 years or above;
- Must be a Singapore citizen;
- Must pass a means the test under the Ministry of Health's Intermediate- and Long-term care (ILTC) non-residential framework;
- Must come from a household where the monthly income per person is $1,800 or below, or the annual value of the residence reflected on the NRIC is $13,000 or below for a household with no income;
- Must be assessed or has been assessed by a qualified assessor (e.g. a therapist, registered nurse, doctor or audiologist) to determine the need and the type of device;
- Must has not have made any previous claim for a similar mobility device.

To apply:

- Seniors currently under the care of a public hospital, community hospital, day rehab centre or senior care centre may approach the therapist or social worker to help with the SMF application.
- Seniors who need to apply for SMF subsidy for hearing aids but are currently not under the care of any hospital will have to get a referral letter from a polyclinic or CHAS clinic for a subsidised hearing assessment at a public hospital. The audiologist will help with the SMF application.
- Seniors who are currently not under the care of a public hospital, community hospital, day rehab centre or senior care centre may download the form https://www.silverpages.sg/sites/silverpagesassets/SilverPages%20Assets/Application%20Forms%20(Financial,%20Care%20Services)/SMF/SMF%20Assistive%20Devices%20Form.pdf or get it from an AICare link office. E-mail or mail the form and required documents to AIC.

Criteria for Transport

To be eligible, the senior:

- Must be a Singapore citizen, aged 60 years or above;
- Must be assessed to need a wheelchair to move around, or need special transport (such as a vehicle with someone who can help him or her get in and out), or rely on walking aids to get around, or need assistance when travelling;

- Must be attending a Ministry of Health–funded eldercare centres (such as a social day care centre, day rehabilitation centre, dementia day care centre or senior care centre), dialysis centre or day hospices;
- Must not be receiving any other subsidy for similar specialised transport services;
- Must pass a means test under the Ministry of Health's ILTC non-residential framework;
- Must come from a household with a monthly income per person of $2,600 or below.

To apply:

Approach the therapist or centre manager of the above-mentioned day care facilities. If the criterion is met, the centre staff will assist you to apply for the subsidy.

Criteria for Home Healthcare Items

To be eligible, the senior:

- Must be a Singapore citizen aged 60 years or above;
- Must be receiving home-based healthcare services such as a home nursing or home medical service, or must be a client of the AIC's Singapore Programme for Integrated Care for the Elderly (SPICE);
- Must not be receiving any other subsidy for similar items;
- Must undergo assessment to determine the need and the type of healthcare items required;
- Must pass a means test under the Ministry of Health's ILTC non-residential framework;
- Must come from a household with a monthly income per person of $1,800 or below.

To apply:

Approach your home healthcare provider — home medical, home nursing or a SPICE centre — about your application for SMF consumables.

Foreign Domestic Worker Levy Concessions

Website: https://www.silverpages.sg/financial-assistance/foreign-domestic-workers/Foreign%20Domestic%20Worker%20(FDW)%20Levy%20Concession

Foreign Domestic Worker (FDW) Levy Concession for Persons with Disabilities

Families who employ full-time FDWs to look after their loved ones with disabilities can pay a lower monthly concessionary FDW levy of $60 (instead of $265) if they are eligible for this scheme.

Each household is eligible for levy concessions for up to two FDWs at any one time, including a concession granted under the other levy concession schemes.*

>*These are the "Young Child/Grandchild" and "Aged Person" levy concession schemes.

To be eligible for the scheme, you will need to meet the following criteria:

(1) *Citizenship*
The care recipient must be a Singapore citizen, aged 16–64 years.

(2) *Medical assessment*
A Singapore-registered doctor must certify that the care recipient needs permanent assistance in at least one activity of daily living (ADL). The six ADLs are:
- Showering/bathing
- Dressing
- Feeding
- Toileting
- Transferring from bed to upright chair/wheelchair, or vice versa
- Moving indoors from room to room on a level surface

Note: This is a non-exhaustive list.

(3) *Relationship with the care recipient*
The FDW employer must be (a) the care recipient or (b) a family member. In the case of (b), the employer and the care recipient must live at the same NRIC-registered address.

Foreign Domestic Worker Levy Concession under Aged Person Scheme

Website: http://www.mom.gov.sg/passes-and-permits/work-permit-for-foreign-domestic-worker/foreign-domestic-worker-levy/levy-concession#-for-aged-persons

Aged Person Scheme (FDW Employer or Spouse)

Eligibility:

- You or your spouse is a Singapore citizen;
- 65 years old or above;
- Living at the same NRIC address as the employer.

If one person is a Singapore citizen and the other is a Singapore Permanent Resident aged 65 years or above, living at the same NRIC address, they will be eligible also.

The concession rate will be given automatically; there is no need to apply.

Aged Person Scheme (Parent or Grandparent)

Eligibility:

- If you or your spouse has a parent, parent-in-law, grandparent or grandparent-in-law who is:

    – A Singapore citizen;
    – Aged 65 years or above;
    – Living at the same NRIC-registered address as you.

- You are also eligible if you or your spouse is a Singapore citizen and the aged person (relationship as defined above) is a Singapore permanent resident aged 65 years or above who lives at the same NRIC-registered address as you.
- You need to apply if you did not give the aged person's information when you applied for an FDW.

Foreign Domestic Worker Grant

Website: https://www.silverpages.sg/financial-assistance/foreign-domestic-workers/Foreign%20Domestic%20Worker%20(FDW)%20Grant

The Foreign Domestic Worker (FDW) Grant is a monthly grant of $120 to support families who need to hire an FDW to care for their loved ones with at least moderate disability.

The grant is applicable only for one FDW per care recipient, capped at two FDWs caring for two care recipients per household at any one time.

You are eligible if you meet all the following criteria:

(1) *Citizenship*

The care recipient is a Singapore citizen or a permanent resident. He or she must be 65 years old or above, and the FDW employer must be a Singapore citizen.

(2) *Relationship to the care recipient*

If you are the FDW employer, the care recipient must be your spouse, parent/parent-in-law, grandparent/grandparent-in-law, child/child-in-law, grandchild/grandchild-in-law or sibling/sibling-in-law.

(3) *Medical assessment*

The care recipient must be assessed by a Singapore-registered doctor. He or she is likely to require permanent assistance in performing at least three of the ADLs:

- Showering/bathing
- Dressing
- Feeding
- Toileting
- Transferring from bed to upright chair/wheelchair, or vice versa
- Moving about on a level floor without help

The doctor will do a functional assessment report, which you must send to the AIC. Contact your preferred doctor before making the visit, to ensure that he or she provides the required assessment service. You can also refer to the list of appointed medical assessors if you are unable to find a suitable doctor.

A medical assessment is not required if the care recipient has any of the following documents:

- Approval letter for ElderShield or Interim Disability Assistance Programme for the Elderly (IDAPE);
- A memo or document from any Singapore-registered doctor certifying that the care recipient is bedridden.

(4) *Household income*

Your household monthly income per person must be $2,600 or less. If your household has no income, the annual value of your property must be less than $13,000.

You do not need to undergo means testing if all members of your household have undergone that in the past two years.

(5) *Caregivers' training*

Your FDW is required to attend the relevant caregiver training course approved by the AIC. Please Select a Caregivers Training Grant (CTG)–approved course from the Caregivers Training Courses e-Calendar. When applying for a course for your FDW so that you can receive the Foreign Domestic Worker Grant, on in the course calendar click on the box entitled "Grant" and select "Yes".

How to apply for the FDW Grant?

(i) Hire an FDW to care for the care recipient;
(ii) Send the FDW for a caregiver training course;
(iii) Submit the household means-testing form to the MOH;
(iv) Prepare the FDW Grant application form and required documents;
(v) Submit them to the AIC.

For a step-by-step guide, refer to the following website: https://www.silverpages.sg/sites/silverpagesassets/SilverPages%20Assets/Application%20Forms%20(Financial,%20Care%20Services)/FAQs%20Screenshots/FDWG/FDWG%20FAQ.pdf

Caregiver Training Grant (CTG)

Website: https://www.silverpages.sg/CTG

This is an annual subsidy for caregivers to attend CTG-approved training courses. A sum of $200 is allocated to each care recipient every financial year (from April to March of the following year). Care recipients must be Singaporeans or permanent residents above the age of 65 or have a disability (as certified by a Singapore-registered doctor).

Family members or foreign domestic workers who are the main caregivers for these care recipients can attend a wide range of CTG-approved courses pertaining to:

- Managing day-to-day care;
- Caring for loved ones with dementia, chronic illnesses, etc.;
- Preventing falls and ensuring home safety;
- Managing loved ones with disability.

Polyclinic Subsidy

Polyclinics provide cheaper rates for Singaporeans and permanent residents of consultations of both medical and dental appointments. Medicines are also subsidised at polyclinics.

Community Health Assist Scheme (CHAS)

Website: https://www.chas.sg/

CHAS is a scheme by the Ministry of Health that enables Singapore citizens from lower- and middle-income households to receive subsidies for medical and dental care at participating general Practitioners and dental clinics near their homes.

Singapore Citizens of all ages are eligible for CHAS if they meet the following criteria:

- Household monthly income per person of $1,800 or below;
- Annual Value of residence as reflected on the NRIC of $21,000 and below for households with no income.

The application form can be obtained from a restructured hospital, polyclinic, community centre club (CC), or Community Development Council (CDC). Alternatively, you can download the form at http://www.chas.sg/templates.aspx?id=196. Only one copy of the form is needed for one household.

Pioneer Generation Package

The term "Pioneer Generation" is defined as living Singaporeans who meet two criteria:

- Aged 16 and above in 1965 (born on or before 31 December 1949, which means that they were aged 65 and above in 2014);
- Obtained citizenship on or before 31 December 1986.

The benefits include:

(1) *Outpatient care*
   - Additional 50% off subsidised services at Specialist Outpatient Clinics (SOCs) and polyclinics;
   - Additional 50% off subsidised medications at SOCs and polyclinics;
   - Subsidies at participating General Practitioners and dental clinics under the Community Health Assist Scheme (CHAS);
   - The Pioneer Generation Disability Assistance Scheme (Pioneer DAS) will provide cash assistance of $1,200 a year to help those with moderate to severe functional disabilities.

(2) *Medisave top-ups*

The Government will provide annual Medisave top-ups of $200–$800 to the pioneer generation, depending on the birth cohort. Those who are older will receive more.

Lifetime Annual Medisave Top-ups for the Pioneer Generation

Age in 2014 (Birth Cohorts)	Amount Per Year
65–69 (1945–1949)	$200
70–74 (1940–1944)	$400
75–79 (1935–1939)	$600
80 and above (1934 and earlier)	$800

(3) *MediShield Life*
   - Support for all pioneers' MediShield Life premiums with special premium subsidies (40%–60%) and Medisave top-ups ($200–$800).
     - Born in 1934 and earlier: Premiums fully covered;
     - Born in 1935–1949 and fully insured under MediShield previously — Pay half the amount of premiums as compared to MediShield.
   - All Pioneers will pay less premiums for MediShield Life than for MediShield.

Pioneer Generation Disability Assistance Scheme (Pioneer DAS)

Website: https://www.silverpages.sg/financial-assistance/Pioneer%20 Generation%20Disability%20Assistance%20Scheme%20%28PioneerDAS%29

    This scheme provides cash assistance of $100 per month to those from the pioneer generation who have moderate to severe functional disabilities, which are defined as requiring assistance for at least three out of the six common ADLs.

    An eligible pioneer was born before 1950 and became a Singapore citizen before 1987, and requires help for at least three ADLs as assessed by a Singaporean doctor. The ADLs are:

- Showering/bathing
- Dressing
- Feeding
- Toileting
- Transferring from bed to upright chair/wheelchair, or vice versa
- Mobility

    The application form for schemes administered by the AIC and the functional assessment form can be obtained from a community centre/club, hospital or polyclinic, or downloaded from the website stated above.

    Eligible pioneers already on ElderShield or IDAPE, or receiving the Foreign Domestic Worker Grant, will not need to undergo this assessment again. Bedridden older persons' application requires only a doctor's note.

CareShield Life

https://www.moh.gov.sg/careshieldlife/about-careshield-life

    The Ministry of Health had recently announced that a new long-term care insurance, CareShield Life, will be launched in 2020.

    This is an improved version of the current Eldershield scheme.

    There will be:

— lifetime cash payouts as long as the patient is unable to do three out of the six ADLs.

— payouts increase over time, depending on which year the claim is started.

Eligibility

- **If you are born in 1980 or later.** If you are born between 1980 to 1990 (aged 30 to 40 in 2020, you will be automatically covered by CareShield Life in 2020. If you are born after 1990 (aged below 30 in 2020), you will be automatically covered by CareShield Life when you turn 30.
- **If you are born in 1979 or earlier.** You can choose to join CareShield Life in 2021, if you are not severely disabled. To make joining CareShield Life more convenient, you will be automatically covered by CareShield Life from 2021 if you are a Singapore Resident born between 1970 and 1979 and are insured under the ElderShield 400 scheme and are not severely disabled. If you are automatically covered and do not wish to participate in the scheme, you have up to 31 Dec 2023 to opt out from the scheme and get your premiums refunded.

Merdeka Generation

PM Lee just announced the new Merdeka Generation package at the National Rally 2018. The Merdeka Generation are Singaporeans born between 1950 and 1959.

The package will cover the following:

- Outpatient subsidies
- MediSave top up
- Medishield Life Premuim Subsidies
- Payouts for long term care
  More information more be available later.

PART 2: LASTING POWER OF ATTORNEY (LPA)

Website: https://www.publicguardian.gov.sg/opg/pages/the-lpa-the-lasting-power-of-attorney.aspx

The lasting power of attorney is a legal document which allows anyone above the age of 21 to voluntarily appoint one or more persons to act and make decisions on his or her behalf if he or she should lose mental capacity one day. It is under the purview of the Office of the Public Guardian of Singapore.

The document is drawn up for those above age 21 with the mental capacity to plan ahead, against the loss of their mental capacity owing to severe illnesses, advanced dementia or traumatic brain injuries from accidents.

Making an LPA is very simple. It involves downloading forms from the Office of the Public Guardian website and making an appointment with an accredited issuer, who can be a physician, lawyer or Singapore Medical Council–registered psychiatrist in Singapore. All the information can be obtained from the website stated.

After obtaining the certification, the person applying for the LPA is to send the application form, certificates and copies of his or her identity card to the Office of the Public Guardian to register.

The LPA form comes in two versions. LPA form 1 is a standard form for health and financial affairs, with basic restrictions on the donee or donees. LPA form 2 will have non-standard requirements that the person may want to include and is done and issued by lawyer.

The LPA is activated when any accredited physician certifies that the person has lost mental capacity and is unable to manage his or her own affairs. The donee or donees can then step forward and make decisions on his or her behalf. Should the person recover mental capacity, he or she will regain the authority to make informed decisions on his or her own.

PART 3: APPOINTMENT OF A DEPUTY FOR AN OLDER PERSON LACKING MENTAL CAPACITY

Website: https://www.familyjusticecourts.gov.sg/Common/Pages/AppointingaDeputy.aspx

A deputy is a person appointed by the court, who is given the authority to make decisions on behalf of a person who lacks mental capacity in relation to his or her personal welfare and/or property and affairs.

For the appointment of deputy, the family of the older person who wish to act legally as his or her proxy decision-maker will have to make an application to the court. The family will have to engage a lawyer to draft all the legal documents for that request. The documents required are:

- Form 217 (Originating Summons)
- Form 218 (Deputy's Affidavit)
- Form 224 (Doctor's Affidavit and Medical Report)
- Form 220 (Consent of Relevant Persons)

Prior to making the court application, the family will have to get the older person's regular physician or a psychiatrist to provide a medical report and a statement that the person is mentally incapable of managing his or her own affairs.

The lawyer will then submit all available documents to the court for their consideration. A date will be set for the case conference and hearings. Not all requests will be approved and it will ultimately be the judge's decision on a case-by-case basis.

PART 4: USEFUL INFORMATION FOR ELDERCARE

Useful websites for getting information:

- http://www.aic.sg
- https://www.silverpages.sg
- Eldercare Services Locator:
  https://www.silverpages.sg/eldercare/searchByServices.aspx?Title=Eldercare%20Locator#.U2cvlPmSx8E
- Information about medical conditions and treatment:
  https://www.singhealth.com.sg/OlderpersonCare/ConditionsAndTreatments/Pages/home.aspx
- Information about drugs and supplements:
  http://www.nlm.nih.gov/medlineplus/druginformation.html

    Useful apps:

- Mobile Eldercare Locator (MEL) from the Agency for Integrated Care
- AICare Link from the Agency for Integrated Care, to find a suitable funding scheme for the care of a dependent elderly person

6 Current and Future Technologies Supporting Eldercare

Singapore has been developing into a smart nation, with multiple initiatives pushing each sector to use technologies to lessen the burden on the manpower requirements, yet improving the efficiency and outcome.

There are many technologies out there in the market for healthcare. To the author, they are grouped into either physical devices/equipment or Internet-of-things platforms facilitating information flow and healthcare service usage.

The potential uses of technology in healthcare and eldercare are endless and can be very broad. Here, they are grouped into various permutations in order to reflect the usefulness and functionality of the technologies, so as, to help save sweat and tears for the caregivers.

TYPES AND USES OF TECHNOLOGIES

The main pointers for the technology can be divided into four main categories, with different permutations of the categories possible when describing that technology:

(1) Who is using the technology? The senior him or herself, the caregiver or the healthcare service provider?
(2) What are the types of deficit to be overcome — physical, sensory neuro or cognitive?
   The types of deficit can be subcategorised into ten different types of deficit, from the author's experience:
   - Physical — paraplegia, meaning that the older person is paralysed from the waist down

- Physical — hemiplegia, meaning that the older person is paralysed from one side of the body, likely from a stroke
- Physical — movement or coordination disorder, a common example being Parkinson's disease
- Physical — amputee (upper or lower limbs)
- Physical — generalised weakness, functional decline, fraility
- Sensory neuro — visual impairment
- Sensory neuro — hearing impairment
- Sensory neuro — tasting impairment
- Sensory neuro — smelling impairment
- Cognitive impairment, e.g. dementia

(3) How do these technologies support the activities of daily living for those in the shadow of these deficits?

The technologies to support these disabling deficits.

- Activity of daily living — transferring
- Activity of daily living — mobility
- Activity of daily living — toileting
- Activity of daily living — bathing
- Activity of daily living — dressing
- Activity of daily living — eating
- Instrumental activity of daily living — shopping
- Instrumental activity of daily living — housekeeping
- Instrumental activity of daily living — accounting (managing finances)
- Instrumental activity of daily living — food/medication preparation
- Instrumental activity of daily living — communication (use of communication devices)
- Instrumental activity of daily living — transportation in community

(4) What are these technologies? A physical device, a mobile application or something with artificial intelligence?

Lastly, we come to the types of technology use, which are here divided into four big groups:

- Physical devices (assistive)
- Physical devices (robotic)
- Physical devices (monitoring)
- IOT platforms

EXAMPLES OF CURRENT NEW TECHNOLOGIES AND FUTURE TECHNOLOGIES

The authors have worked on multiple technologies in the past and present, in the course of their work. Here are some of the various technologies that can be used in the near future.

Exoskeleton

We now have new devices such as the exoskeleton to replace older ones, like the wheelchair or the walking frame. There are quite a few products out in the market, and many are still in the trial phase and not commercially available yet in Singapore. One such product is from ExoAtlet Asia. The advantages of using exoskeletal robotics include:

- Getting the joy of walking upright again and talking to everyone at face-to-face level;

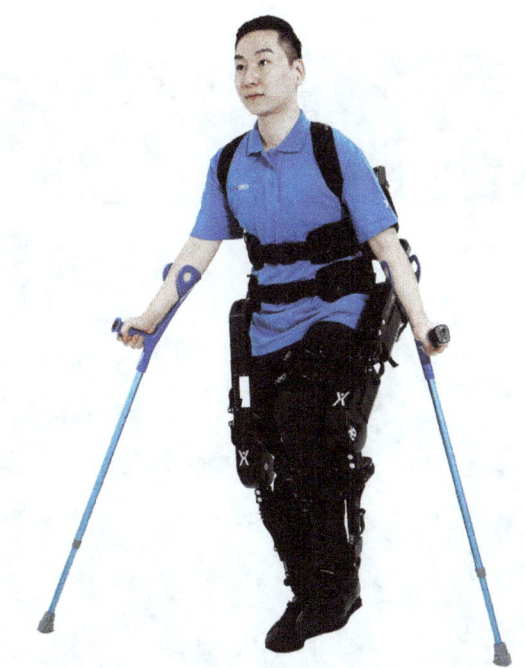

- Improving the function of a previously wheelchair-bound older person with endless possibilities of the newfound freedom off the wheelchair;
- Improving upright posture bodily functions, such as promoting gastro-intestinal movement and relieving constipation;
- Potentially reducing the incidence of bedsores and the risk of osteoporosis, besides many other proven health benefits;
- Improving self-esteem from standing upright again;
- Enabling more social interactions amongst PWDs using our robots — similar to car clubs for improving social interactions. They can be the star at in social events, with many interesting stories about the use of exoskeleton robotics.

Telemonitoring, Teleconsultations and Telepresence Devices

Both the older person and the caregiver can be isolated and, at times, to take an elderly person to hospital may involve a lot of effort and

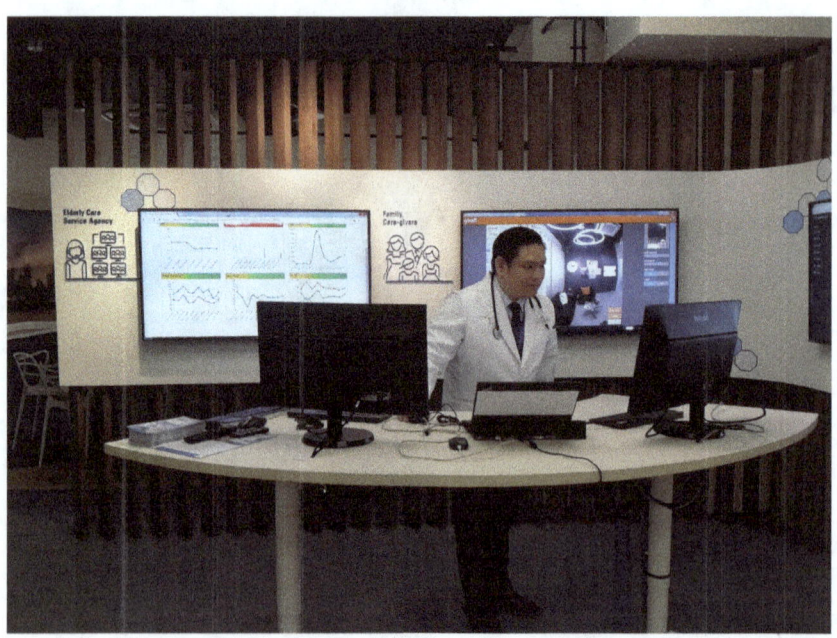

resources. Teleconsultations, remote monitoring and telepresence can be very useful now and in the near future for facilitating efficient and convenient reviews.

Telemonitoring

What are the possible current remote monitoring devices?

- Remote blood pressure monitoring through a Bluetooth-enabled automated blood pressure meter;
- Remote heart rate monitoring through either a Bluetooth-enabled automated blood pressure meter or a pulse oximeter;
- Remote blood oxygen saturation monitoring through a Bluetooth-enabled pulse oximeter;
- Remote respiratory rate monitoring through a Bluetooth-enabled bed monitoring mat;
- Remote capillary glucose monitoring through a Bluetooth-enabled blood glucometer.

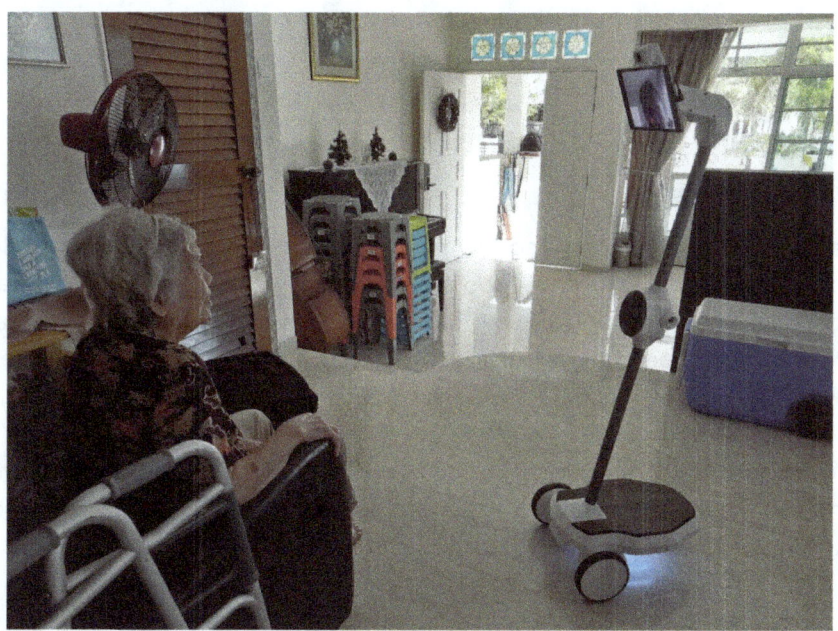

Telepresence robot from OhmniLabs.

Teleconsultations

Teleconsultations can be made possible by using a telepresence robot at home with certain telehealth equipment such as a Bluetooth enabled stethoscope or dermoscope.

Teleprescription

In future, with the availability of the National Electronic Health Records and the compulsory use of electronic medical records, teleprescribing at a teleconsultation session will be very possible. There are already teleprescription platforms available for use.

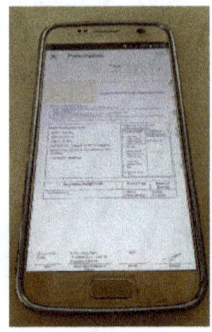

Telewound

Telewound services can also be made possible in future, using mobile applications to measure wounds and chart the wound recovery or deterioration. The application being incorporated with artificial intelligence, the wound can be managed remotely. The caregiver will be supported by a wound care nurse using the teleconsultation platforms via telepresence equipment.

That will save many trips and logistic nightmares for the older persons and their families. It will also increase the efficiency of the home care wound nurse, saving on travelling time and costs.

We have a local Singaporean company, Nucleus Dynamics, developing such solutions with one of its flagship products, NDKare.

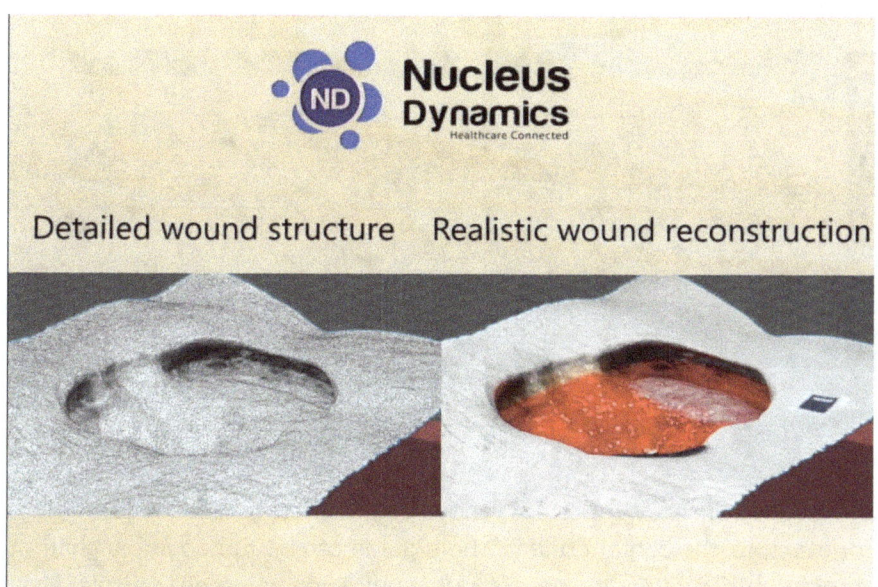

Chatbots

Chatbots have been in use for a long time. Some companies now provide a platform where you can customise your own chatbot. For example, Pastel Health, a France based health technology company, has provided a chatbot platform for healthcare. On the platform, people with no coding background can fully customise a chatbot themselves in whichever language they prefer and the content that they can think of. There are a number of new initiatives in the pipeline to use chatbots to assist both older persons and their caregivers in the near future.

The Chatbots for health website is www.chatbotsforhealth.com

One good example of such chatbots is an experimental chatbot which seniors with cognitive impairment can use to chat. It is like a 24/7 personal assistant to remind the seniors about their families and schedules and, essentially, all their memories. Such chatbots are customised for each individual with very personalised details and content.

Newer chatbots to guide caregivers on processes or procedures will also be out in the near future, giving caregivers a cheap, fast and efficient

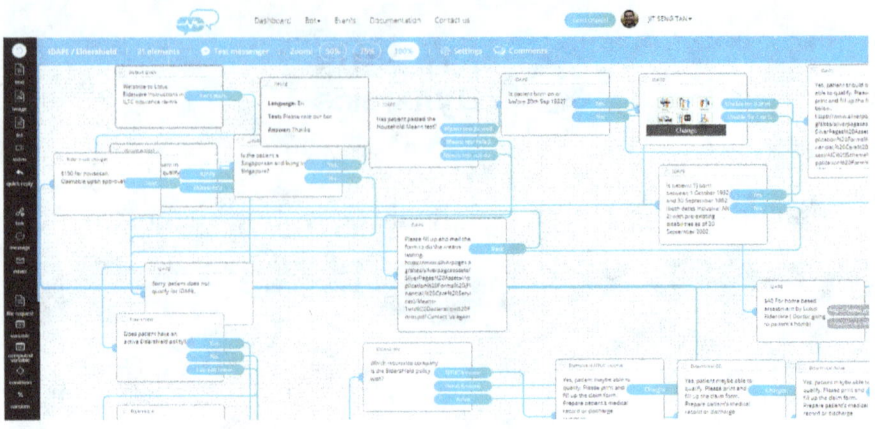

24/7 avenue to seek support for various potential issues faced in caregiving. For example, the content of this whole guide can be turned into a chatbot program and caregivers can get quick guidance when needed 24/7 via chatting on their mobile devices.

Index

Activities Of Daily Living (ADL), 2, 3, 69–71, 75, 77, 81, 86
advance care planning, 62
AeroChamber, 36
air mattress, 34
ambulation, 20
appointment of a deputy, 83

barrier cream, 6, 13
bedpan, 34
bedsores, 42
blended diet, 10
blood capillary glucose, 25
blood pressure chart, 22
blood pressure monitoring, 21, 22
breathless, 54
breathlessness, 46, 53, 55

cardiovascular system, 49
caregiver stress, 61, 67
caregiver training grant, 78
chatbots, 91
chest infections, 47, 51, 52, 54
chest physiotherapy, 39, 52
commode, 34, 35
community health assist scheme, 79
constipation, 48, 49, 52, 55, 58
crutches, 17

delirium, 46, 47, 52, 54, 55
dementia, 58, 64, 79, 83, 86
dentition, 49
depression, 33, 58, 63
diabetes, 30

diabetes mellitus, 55
diapers, 13
dressing, 2, 8, 69, 71, 75, 77, 81, 86
dual-purpose umbrella and walking stick, 17
dyslipidaemia, 56

ear drops, 28
earwax, 57
EASE, 71
endocrine system, 49
epilepsy, 33, 59
evening primrose oil, 33
exoskeleton, 87
eye diseases, 57
eye drops, 27
eye ointment/eye gel, 28

fish oil, 33
foreign domestic worker (FDW) levy, 75
foreign domestic worker grant, 76
full shower or tub bath, 6

gastrointestinal system, 49
Ginkgo biloba, 32
glucosamine, 32
gout, 31, 57

haematological system, 50
hand washing, 5
hearing impairment, 57
heart diseases, 56
heart failure, 54, 55

herpes zoster infection, 53
home care, 63
honey-thickened fluid, 9
hospice, 64
hospital bed, 34
hydraulic lift, 38
hypertension, 31, 56, 65

IDAPE, 69
interim care, 62

lasting power of attorney, 82
liver failure, 55
loss of weight, 51

minced diet, 10
monitoring of weight, 24, 54, 55
musculoskeletal system, 50

nail care, 6
nails, 7
nasogastric tube feeding, 10, 51, 58, 62
nasogastric tube (NGT), 29
nebuliser, 36, 54
nectar-thickened fluid, 9

oral feeding, 9
oral hygiene, 7
oral medications, 27
oxygen concentrator, 35, 36

palliative care, 53
Panax ginseng, 33
Parkinsonism, 58
partial bed bath, 5
passive physiotherapy, 39, 58
percutaneous endoscopic gastrostomy (PEG) tube feeding, 12
performing shaving, 6
perineal hygiene, 14

personal protective equipment, 40
physiotherapy, 58
pioneer generation diability assistance scheme, 81
pioneer generation package, 79
preparing fluids of different consistencies, 9
preparing solids of different consistencies, 10
pudding-thickened fluid, 9
pulmonary tuberculosis, 52
pulse oximetry, 24
pulse rate, 23

QaneMate, 18
quad cane, 17

renal failure, 54
renal system, 50
respiratory failure, 54
respiratory rate, 23
respiratory system, 50
respite care, 61–63
rollator, 18

seizures, 32, 33, 59
sensory system, 51
sitting, 15
skin, 13, 21, 30, 43, 51
skin infection, 53
SMF, 72
soft diet, 10
special diets, 30
stroke, 58, 59, 65
suction machine, 37
supplements, 32
suppository, 48

telemonitoring, 88, 89
telewound, 90
thermometer, 23

Index

transferring, 2, 15, 16, 57, 69, 71, 75, 77, 81, 86
transition of care, 66
transitional care, 62, 65
turning, 9, 12, 15

up from a lying position, 15
urinary catheters, 13
urinary tract infection, 47, 52, 59
urine bags, 13

walking aids, 17
walking frame, 18, 87
walking stick, 17
weight, 54
weight and height, 51
weight loss, 52, 63
wheelator, 19
wheelchair, 19, 87, 88
wound care, 43
wound management, 42

www.ingramcontent.com/pod-product-compliance
Lightning Source LLC
Chambersburg PA
CBHW061944220426
43662CB00012B/2020